Body & Soul

A Girl's Guide to a Fit, Fun, and Fabulous Life

Bethany Hamilton with Dustin Dillberg L.Ac., PAS

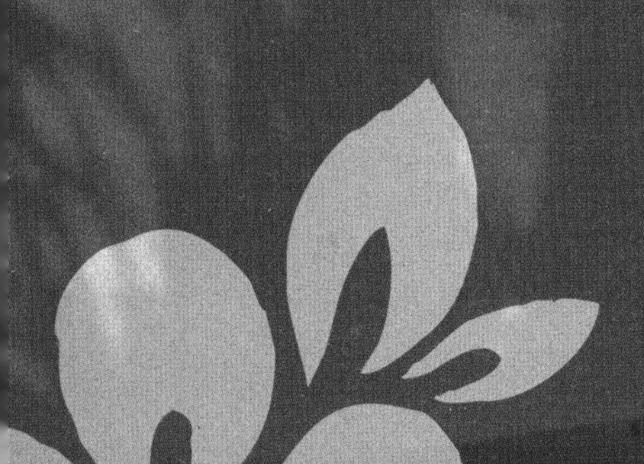

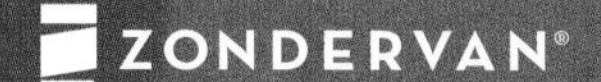

ZONDERVAN

Body and Soul

ISBN: 978-0-310-73105-4

Requests for information should be addressed to:
Zondervan, *3900 Sparks Drive SE., Grand Rapids, Michigan 49546*

Done in association with Red Engine, Baltimore, Maryland

Editors: Kim Childress and Karen Bokram
Cover design: Chun Kim
Interior design: Kris Nelson and Chun Kim
Photography: Sean Scheidt; Noah Hamilton; © tim-mckenna.com
Hair & makeup: Leah Bassett
Styling: Jessica D'Argenio Waller
Produced by: Karen Bokram

Bethany's clothing courtesy of Rip Curl, Under Armour, PrAna. Other clothing courtesy of O'Neill, Under Armour. Jewelry provided by The Knotty Mermaid.

Printed in China

14 15 16 /DSC/ 10 9 8 7 6 5 4 3 2 1

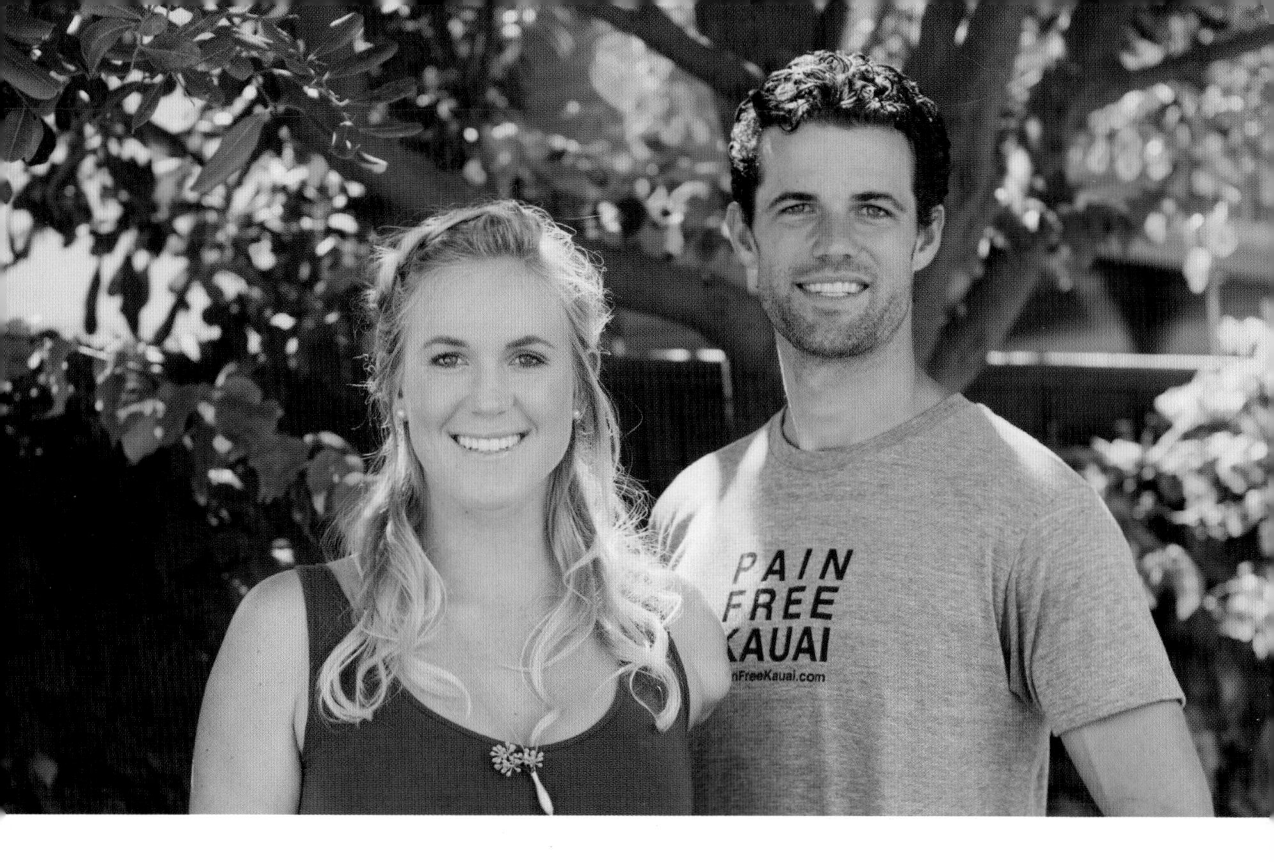

Congratulations!

You've just made an important choice that I believe can change your life. This book you are holding not only contains pages of fun workouts and tasty, good-for-you recipes, it's the starting point for a deeper understanding of how rewarding a fit and healthy lifestyle can be—a lifestyle we have been blessed enough to discover and continue to enjoy. As Dustin's mother used to say, "Luck is when preparation meets opportunity." You're "lucky" when you prepare yourself to seize all the opportunities God has blessed you with. You'll also meet people like Adam (Bethany's husband) and Kirby (our go-to health guru). We hope this book helps you find your healthiest life, your stoked moments, and capture your many God-given blessings and above all a deeper desire to know and live life for God!

Bethany Dustin Dillberg

Bethany Hamilton and Dustin Dillberg

Other books featuring

Bethany Hamilton

Soul Surfer Series Fiction

Clash (Book One)

Burned (Book Two)

Storm (Book Three)

Crunch (Book Four)

• • • • • •

Soul Surfer Series Nonfiction

Ask Bethany

Rise Above, A 90-Day Devotional

I feel blessed with so many things right now ...

like the ability to grow in the knowledge of God's love and the life he calls us to live through him, and the understanding of how to be an overall healthier person. There is so much I've already learned throughout my journey, and I'm grateful to be able to share it all with you in the chapters you are about to read.

There have been numerous people in my life who have taught and encouraged me in my quest to better understand my body.

First, I'd like to thank my parents. They're the ones who encouraged my love for surfing right from the start. Not only that, but both made it possible to choose healthy foods in my diet and work with some awesome trainers.

I'd like to thank my sister-in-law for showing great work ethic and helping me translate my thoughts to paper. Thanks for always seeking the Lord; his love shows in your life! I feel very blessed to work with you and have you as my sister.

I'd also like to thank Dustin and Kirby Dillberg and the Dillberg ohana for educating and encouraging me so much throughout the years. Dustin, your expertise is RAD. Let the learning journey continue!

To my husband, Adam: Thanks for your willingness to always try my delicious (and sometimes crazy!) healthy recipes and for all of the fun we've had so far in the kitchen. Mahalo for running the deep sand beaches and killer hills with the dogs and me. But most of all, thank you for loving me like Jesus loves me.

—BH

TABLE OF CONTENTS

Get More Out of *Body & Soul!*

This book features multimedia content beyond the printed page.

Some of the pages in this edition of *Body & Soul* feature special icons you can use to activate and discover additional content on your smartphone, mobile, or tablet device.

HOW DOES IT WORK?

1.  Visit the app store to download the free HarperCollins Unbound app for your iOS, Android, or Windows mobile device.
2. When you see this icon on the pages throughout the book, open the app on your device and scan the page.
3. The app will do the rest, bringing multimedia and interactive content that relates to the page you're reading right into your device.

For additional information visit: www.harpercollinsunbound.com.

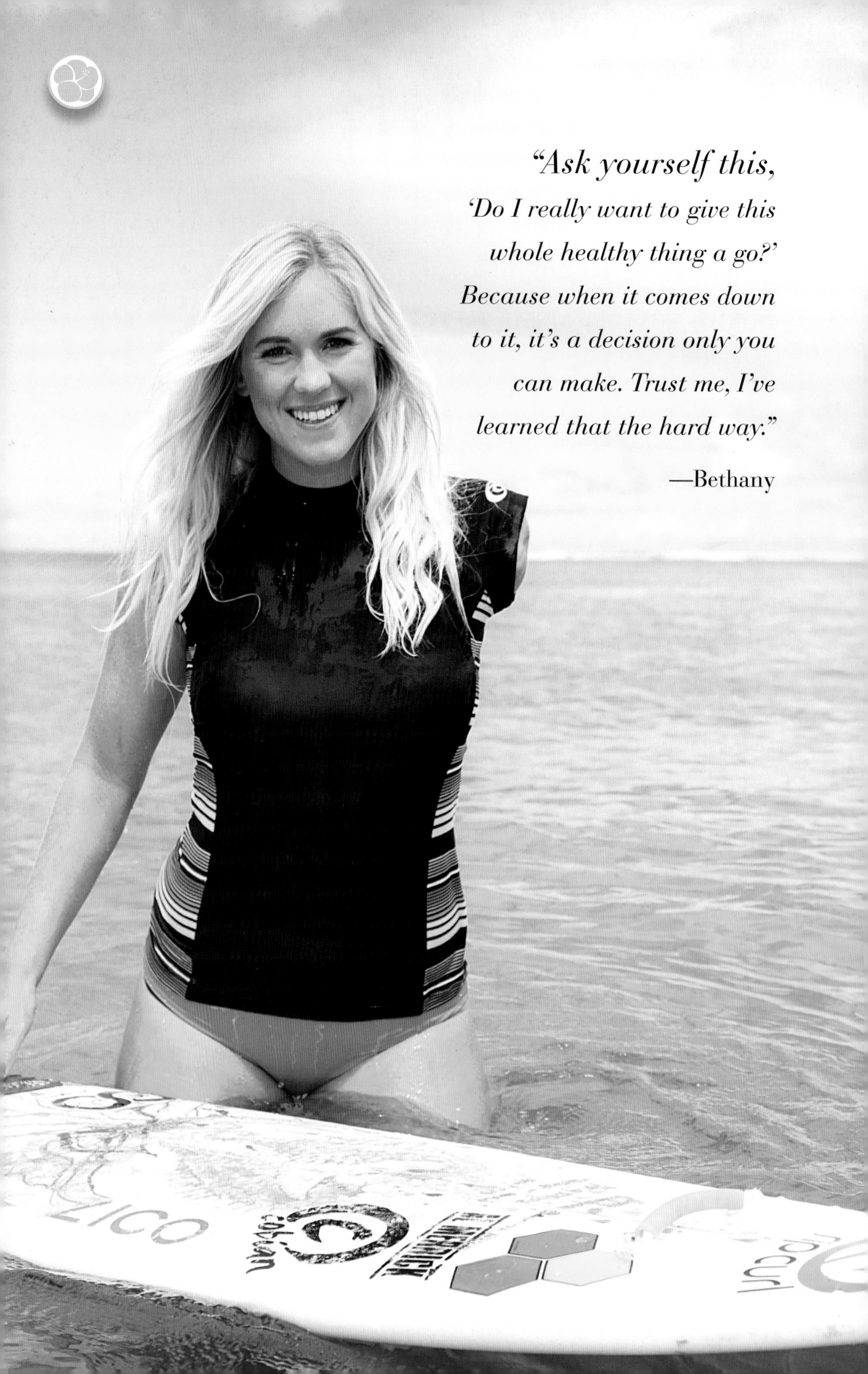
"Ask yourself this,
'Do I really want to give this
whole healthy thing a go?'
Because when it comes down
to it, it's a decision only you
can make. Trust me, I've
learned that the hard way."
—Bethany

CHAPTER 1

In Total Confidence

Picture yourself slipping into the water, the waves brushing against your legs. Everything that's going on in your life, all your worries and stress, just melt away as you step up on that board and glide across the water's surface. Catching the best wave you can find, with each wave unique from the wave before. No matter how good or bad a session you might have, you're having fun doing what you love, enjoying God's beautiful creation and just being yourself ... every single day. This is why I love surfing.

I began catching waves when I was a toddler. I was literally learning to surf and walk at the same time. I guess growing up in a house of ocean lovers will do that to you. Without a doubt, one of the first things surfing taught me was dedication.

Let's start with my parents. If I didn't have dedicated parents willing to sacrifice so much to take me to the beach every day (and not just because they wanted to zap the energy out of me and my brothers, Timmy and Noah, so we'd be mellow at night, although I like to joke that was part of it), I wouldn't have gotten to where I am now.

I would go to surf competitions just about every other weekend. Even the little keiki surf contests my parents signed me up for when I was five showed me the importance of sticking to something you love. And I wouldn't let anything strip me of that dedication, not even losing my left arm to a fourteen-foot tiger shark when I was thirteen.

As you might have noticed, I'm missing a piece of my body (hello, stating the obvious!). But it's not a big deal, really. And even though I look different than most people, one arm is the normal me; it's become a part of who I am. And the great thing is, I'm loved by God, one arm and all.

If you're not familiar with my story, here's what happened: On October 31, 2003, a shark attacked me while I was surfing off the north shore of Kauai. I lost over 60 percent of my blood and almost lost my life.

I faced two very intense surgeries and was in the hospital for about a week. My life definitely came to a screeching halt that scary morning. I had a lot to face. But with God's help, my hope in him, and the passions he has given me, I came out of this one-armed—and determined. I was willing to stop at nothing to get back in the water and continue doing what I enjoyed. A month after the attack, that's what I did.

And now I've been a professional surfer since I was seventeen. I work hard at the sport I adore. Working hard and having fun has helped me take everything I've learned and apply it to other areas of my life—most importantly, a rewarding, healthy lifestyle.

The changes I've made not only help me with my athletic performance, they've left me feeling incredible. Sure, I still have a lot to learn in my own journey, but the tidbits I have picked up and tested along the way are things I think everyone should try out.

You don't need to drop a lot of money, spend hours and hours in the gym or give up the foods you enjoy (mmm, chocolate!) to feel—and look—amazing.

And no, you don't have to be a pro athlete to get there either. (Of course, if you've developed some unhealthy eating habits, like frequent binges on chips or ice cream, you may have to find some substitutes, which this book will help you do.)

Being in a good place with your fitness and eating habits will put you in a good place to face other things throughout your days, months, and years.

And it's not just about working out or eating right that'll help you get the results you want. Learning to love God and discovering what it means to live for him will help too. Being healthy overall—physically and spiritually—are steps to feeling fabulous.

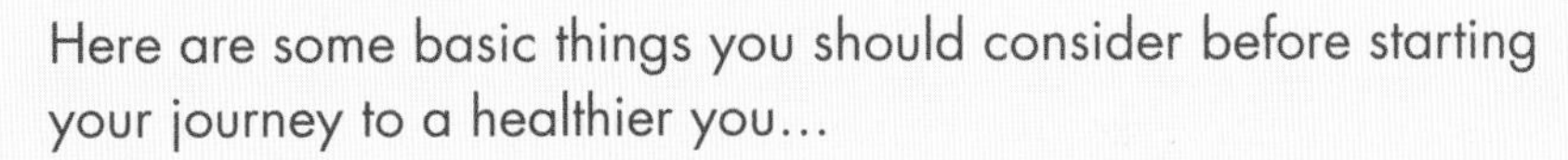

ARE YOU READY FOR CHANGE?

Here are some basic things you should consider before starting your journey to a healthier you...

* Do you want to improve your overall health and look better within your body's limits?
* Are you willing to not let any negative talk slow you down or keep you from your goals?
* Are you up for trying a new workout, a new sport, or healthy food (within your means) at least once?
* Are you OK with keeping a positive mindset no matter what the day brings?
* Do you trust that God's love for you will help you along your journey?

Anybody can achieve a fulfilling, soulful life. But you've gotta promise me one thing: Don't focus on being me, Bethany Hamilton (though I hope you'll find a lot of inspiration in the things I'm about to share with you). Focus on working towards being the best, beautiful inside-and-out, unique, rad *you,* because that's really what it's all about. Are you ready?

THE PLUNGE

Ask yourself this: Do I *really* want to give this whole healthy thing a go? Because when it comes down to it, it's a decision only *you* can make. Trust me, I've learned that the hard way. I used to try to make my mom eat healthy, and let's just say, it didn't work at all. I've tried to get my brother Noah to work out with me but eventually realized what he really likes to do is surf, so we stick to doing that together.

No matter how much I want *others* to make improvements to their lifestyles, I can't push them to make a change. But *you* have all the power to push yourself, and the best part is that *you* already have all of the tools.

OK, I'll admit I wasn't really dedicated to eating super healthy when I was younger. Butterfingers were definitely my go-to. *Eek!* A lot of athletes will just eat whatever junk food they want. And since they're constantly burning calories with practice, they think they can get away with it. But almost all of the time it catches up eventually in some form or another.

The more I started educating myself on nutritious foods, the more I realized that it was only a matter of time before my bad eating habits would catch up with me.

The truth is, you may look fine and healthy on the outside, but your body is not guaranteed to be very healthy inside if you're not giving it the proper fuel.

I guess my "aha" moment of how valuable it is to take your health into your own hands came during my late teens. I got my period when I was thirteen, but stopped getting it shortly after—a common occurence among female athletes, often caused by a combination of too much exercise, too few calories, and too much stress on the body due to training.

I know what you're thinking. No cramps? No leaks? Sign me up! But not having a normal cycle actually isn't good for you. So by the time I was seventeen, I decided to change all of that.

After going to a health care specialist to devise a plan, I kicked off a month-long cleanse of eating clean foods (as in nothing processed or refined), lots of veggies and herbal supplements given to me by my doc. Eventually, my periods returned (phew!), and I discovered how powerful eating right can be. My energy levels also improved and I was actually becoming a *woman*. Woo-hoo!

Of course, the whole idea of changing my diet was overwhelming at first, but I quickly learned you just need discipline.

I'm the type of person who loves soaking up information and learning from others. Working with someone who clearly spent his whole life studying the human body gave me this desire to give what he said a go. And once I saw I could improve something about myself naturally by really thinking through everything that goes into my body, it encouraged me to improve even more elements of my health.

YOUR BLUEPRINT FOR SUCCESS

Pause for a second. Hold out your palms and take a close look at them, creases and all. Glance down at your feet and flex them both. Step in front of a mirror and stare at your reflection. Everything that you see, God planned specifically for you before you were even born.

It's easy to get caught up in all of the negative things we don't like about our bodies. I find that we as girls, especially, compare ourselves to others. Instead of comparing or complaining, take time to appreciate what you have, the good in you and others, and most of all, how God has created the uniqueness of Y-O-U.

Negative thinking is only going to hold you back from understanding how powerful your body actually is. Instead of dwelling on what you might not have, it's essential to focus on being thankful for what you've been given.

For you created my inmost being; you knit me together in my mother's womb. I praise you because I am fearfully and wonderfully made; your works are wonderful, I know that full well. My frame was not hidden from you when I was made in the secret place, when I was woven together in the depths of the earth. Your eyes saw my unformed body; all the days ordained for me were written in your book before one of them came to be.

—PSALM 139:13-16

Not only is each of us unique because God intended it that way, but we're already equipped with the perfect design because of him. He is completely aware of our physical limits.

The point of a healthy lifestyle is getting to the place where you know how to use everything you've been given to its fullest potential. You start to understand all of the beauty and functionality God has placed within you when he created you.

Take a simple stretch, for example. When you bend down, you might only be able to go as far as halfway along your legs at first. But work at it, and you'll soon find you can touch those toes after all.

You might not think your body can physically carry you through a five-mile run, but push yourself and you'll see your body adapt as you pass every mile mark.

When you first do a plank, you might feel like you're gonna die after twenty seconds but as you keep doing it, you'll build yourself up to hold the position for a minute or longer. Trust me, it makes you stoked!

What I'm trying to say is, when you see what your body is capable of achieving when you challenge it, it's all the encouragement you need. So instead of lounging on the couch, lace up those sneakers and start figuring out all of the amazing ways your body can move. I guarantee you'll be surprised by what you discover.

BELIEVE IN THE BENEFITS

When people hear the word healthy, they tend to automatically assume their denim size should be dropping or the reading on the scale should plummet. But you can't measure a fit lifestyle by the numbers, only by the actions you take every day.

When you treat your body better, your body functions better. It's not about what you look like coming out of this, but how you feel. So let's start thinking about the awesome things that come out of just a little hard work and self-love.

One of the biggest benefits I've scored since starting my health journey? A surge in energy. After a few days of not eating well or exercising enough, I feel my energy go down. And the great thing is, you can almost see an instant boost in energy when you start working out and eating right.

OK, I know it's confusing. You might be asking, "Don't you *use* energy to exercise, making you more tired?" Well, yes, you do need energy to push through those lunges or a few reps of wall sits. But instead of losing it in the process, you're actually gaining a ton more. I'll give it to you in technical terms.

Every time you go out for a swim, hop on your bike, or do any sort of exercise for that matter, there's a boost in circulation and blood flow. Blood flow helps deliver more oxygen throughout our bodies, which in turn helps create more energy. Eating right has similar effects. The right fuel at the right time and in the right amount will give you the proper power to make it through the day.

Healthy living is a brain booster too. You know those "feel-good" chemicals you hear a lot about? Just a li'l bit of exercise will get those pumping. Working out ups things that your body naturally produces like dopamine, serotonin, and endorphins, which help regulate stress hormones and anxiety, allowing you better focus. And did I mention you feel amazing because of that flow of endorphins?

FIND THAT CONFIDENCE

Of course you're going to see some physical changes. You might notice a gain in muscle tone. Your skin might clear up, giving off a stunning glow, which lends to a mental boost too. You can look at gaining a healthy lifestyle as also gaining mental confidence.

Say, for example, you do twenty squats a day for a week and then you start thinking, "Oh, this is getting easier—I'm gonna do thirty-five squats a day next week." You're building your body up by amping your routine. But at the same time, you're gaining confidence by noticing your body is getting stronger.

I have a friend who really wants to be a pro surfer. She's super talented, but wouldn't do anything beyond running or biking, neither of which are technically the best training for surfing. Eventually, she started getting in proper strength training and cardio workouts every day. It was awesome to watch her get stronger and to see her confidence soar, which improved her surfing a ton.

Even if you're not trying to go pro, when you do a certain workout move consistently and you feel your body getting better at it, there's something about accomplishing it that makes you feel really good inside. It's a fun, personal challenge, and it can be an awesome thing to do with friends.

Seeing positive results when you continually challenge your body will put you into an upward spiral. And the self-esteem you get from any type of workout will keep energizing you from the inside out—something you can carry into other areas of your life like school, relationships, even extracurricular activities.

It's easy to lose sight of that confidence at times, for sure. I'm not gonna lie, sometimes it's not easy for me.

Right after the attack, I'd get discouraged—and there were some tears. I basically went from this invincible little girl to someone who had to pretty much re-learn everything she had already worked so hard for.

The teenage years were tough for me too. I had just lost my arm, and now the rest of me was changing. It was a lot to take on at once. I had to accept it and realize I could adapt. Once I did, I was able to feel at ease with all the changes.

You can be beautiful no matter what your teen years throw at you. Finding that balance of knowing God, taking care of the body you've been given, and making good decisions as you're growing up into an adult will ensure that.

I'm going to be honest: You're going to face challenges in your day-to-day life—some small and some big. It's how you choose to handle those hurdles that determines how successful you'll be at reaching your goals. So be sure to stand up to the obstacles that come your way rather than let them defeat you. Keep it positive!

Like with most things, the more time you put into it, the closer you'll get to achieving your goals. You can't expect things to just happen—you have to work at it. As my fitness and nutrition trainers, Dustin and Kirby Dillberg (whom you'll be hearing a lot more from in this book) like to say, you should always have the mindset of being better today than you were yesterday.

To get started on a promising, healthy future, you have to commit to make choices starting right now that will improve all of your tomorrows (we'll be sharing those choices later in the book). Be aware that every choice you make in your life counts. It might seem daunting at first, but know that you have the support and encouragement of family, friends, and even me along the way.

I can't stress enough how good I feel when I'm loving God, I'm fit and strong, and I'm making positive choices. That feeling is something I wouldn't want to live without—and I know you will get to the point where you'll feel the same.

It's important to know what makes you feel beautiful and healthy. These can be your "go-to" things to help you push yourself up and off the couch and on the right track again.

THE FIVE THINGS THAT MAKE ME FEEL BEAUTIFUL

- **SURFING.** Coming in from a good session, I feel confident knowing I did well and got an awesome workout. I always come in hungry for more.
- **EATING HEALTHY THROUGHOUT THE DAY.** There's something about good-for-you foods that make you feel great. I mean, who feels beautiful after a pigout? Am I right?
- **GETTING OUTSIDE AND EXERCISING.** I feel so awesome after a workout, especially when I get to enjoy the beautiful surroundings God has given us.
- **STRAIGHT UP LAUGHTER.** When you're laughing a lot, it brings that feeling of joy. And when you're joyful, you feel amazing about yourself and the people around you.
- **MY BFF-TURNED-HUBBY, ADAM.** His love for me no matter what mood I'm in makes me feel great. He really cares for me and takes note of what I like.

Write down five things that make YOU feel beautiful.

1. ....
2. ....
3. ....
4. ....
5. ....

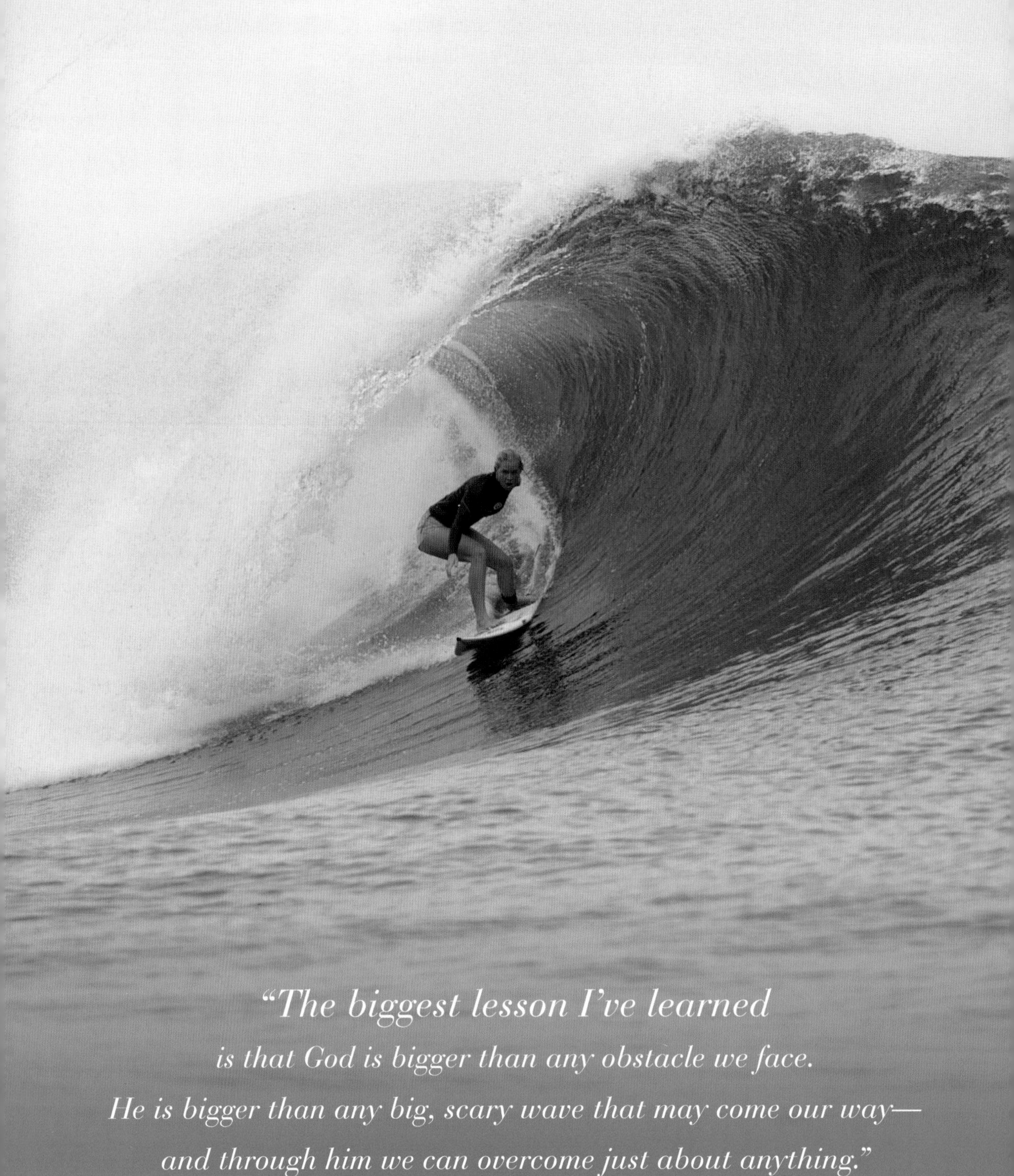

"The biggest lesson I've learned
is that God is bigger than any obstacle we face.
He is bigger than any big, scary wave that may come our way—
and through him we can overcome just about anything."

–Bethany

CHAPTER 2

Your Body Is a Gift

Your body is unique and special. The Bible says "God created man (and woman) in his own image ..." We have incredible bodies that resemble the one who created us. I find that really cool to think about. No doubt, though, my body is different. And because of that, I face challenges every single day. But truthfully, I'm happy with the way I am. I'm able to surf. I'm able to hang out with my friends, run on the beach, and I love to rock my surf gear. Don't get me wrong, there are times when I feel discouraged and not crazy about the way I look. But this is the body I've been given by God, and I cherish it.

Each and every day, I try to glorify God in my body. Whether it's by eating an organic diet, working out, or being a positive role model for other girls who may struggle with body image issues, I'm serving God. The Bible says, "So whether you eat or drink or whatever you do, do it all for the glory of God" (1 Corinthians 10:31).

This verse reminds me that whatever I'm doing—whether it be surfing, running, or goofing off with my BFF—I should do it wholeheartedly for God.

Of course, we all slip here and there. I definitely do. There are days when I'm tempted to eat the junk food around me like chocolate peanut butter cups or skip a workout when I just don't feel like getting out of bed. And there's absolutely nothing wrong with cheating once in a while. But if you make a habit of being unhealthy, it can lead to lots of different health problems.

Do you not know that your bodies are temples of the Holy Spirit, who is in you, whom you have received from God? You are not your own; you were bought at a price. Therefore honor God with your bodies.

1 CORINTHIANS 6:19-20

So how can you glorify God in your body? By first receiving Christ and accepting his love, then asking him to guide you on the path he's laid out for you. It's an awesome adventure!

A MASTER PLAN

It's crazy to think back to when I first asked God into my heart. I was just five years old, sitting in my living room with my best friend, Noelani, when we prayed a simple prayer asking God into our hearts. That was the moment I put my trust in Jesus Christ.

As I got older and more involved with my youth group, and through reading the Bible, I began to understand God more. I realized I wanted to live for him. I invited him to be with me every single second of the day. And why wouldn't I? No matter what I do, he loves me, which is such a beautiful thing.

I believe God has a rad master plan for everyone. You may find this hard to believe, but I think God knew exactly what he was allowing when the shark took my arm.

In fact, just two weeks prior to that fateful October day, my mom and I prayed he'd guide me to be more than just a surfer—I wanted him to spread his light and love through me in a unique way.

I'd just placed second in a huge surfing event with girls way older than me. I was totally stoked, but at the same time, I knew there was another reason I was on earth to honor God in my life. So my mom and I prayed every day he'd show us a way for me to honor him.

Then I lost my arm. And even though I was in the hospital just barely surviving, my mom and I had this sense of peace that God was in control. Though it was a little crazy—and though I couldn't fully see the bigger plan he had—I knew he was in control and would take care of me and my family.

Every day, I spent time talking to Christ. I had this relationship with him. I could trust in him and have faith he would carry me through anything I had to overcome. And he definitely did.

It's awe-inspiring to look back on the experience and see how good God has been in my life. How he can take what seems like something so awful and turn it into something so beautiful? As a pro surfer and motivational speaker, I get to share my story with people all over the world and, more importantly, to share Jesus Christ and his love.

The biggest lesson I've learned is that God is bigger than any obstacle we face. He is bigger than any big, scary wave that may come our way—and through him we can overcome just about anything.

CHERISHING YOUR GIFT

My story may be unique, but even if your biggest challenge is simply getting through a stressful day, know that God is always there for you too. All you have to do is accept that he loves you and that he'll steer you to do what's right. It's such a relief to be able to put your trust in God and take that weight off your shoulders.

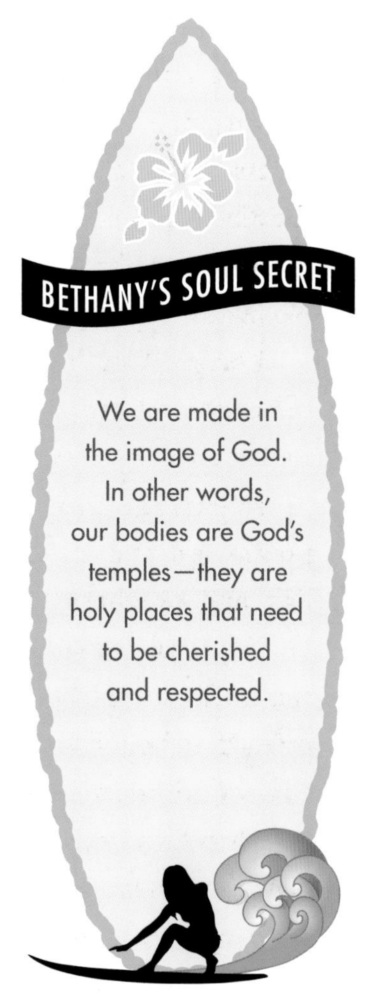

Take my yoke upon you and learn from me,
for I am gentle and humble in heart,
and you will find rest for your souls.
For my yoke is easy and my burden is light.
MATTHEW 11:29-30

And once you accept God's love? It's all about honoring him however you can. Honoring God gives us purpose to live. We are here to make him smile and bring him glory. That glory can be found even in the small things like encouraging one another, not complaining, and even turning off the TV and reading your Bible instead.

A huge part of my relationship with God is treating my body right. After all, we are made in the image of God and his Spirit lives inside us.

Eating right, exercising, and staying healthy are all ways we can honor our "temples." I always say, "Love God, love others, and love yourself."

And when you're in that state of mind, it can encourage you to push through days when you don't want to work out or eat healthy.

Any way you can take care of your body is a way to show God the love and respect you have for him.

You may be thinking, "I just scarfed down a bacon cheeseburger with fries for lunch ... does that mean I'm not respecting God?" Not exactly. God loves you no matter what.

But he also calls on us to be good stewards of our bodies and expects us to protect and feed them properly.

So if you make a habit of hitting up fast food joints every day or sitting around texting instead of exercising, it's probably time for a happy, healthy change.

There are so many things in life we can't control, but we can choose to eat healthy, exercise, and stay positive. That stuff makes a huge difference, from the way you look and feel to how confident you are. And having faith in God makes it all easier.

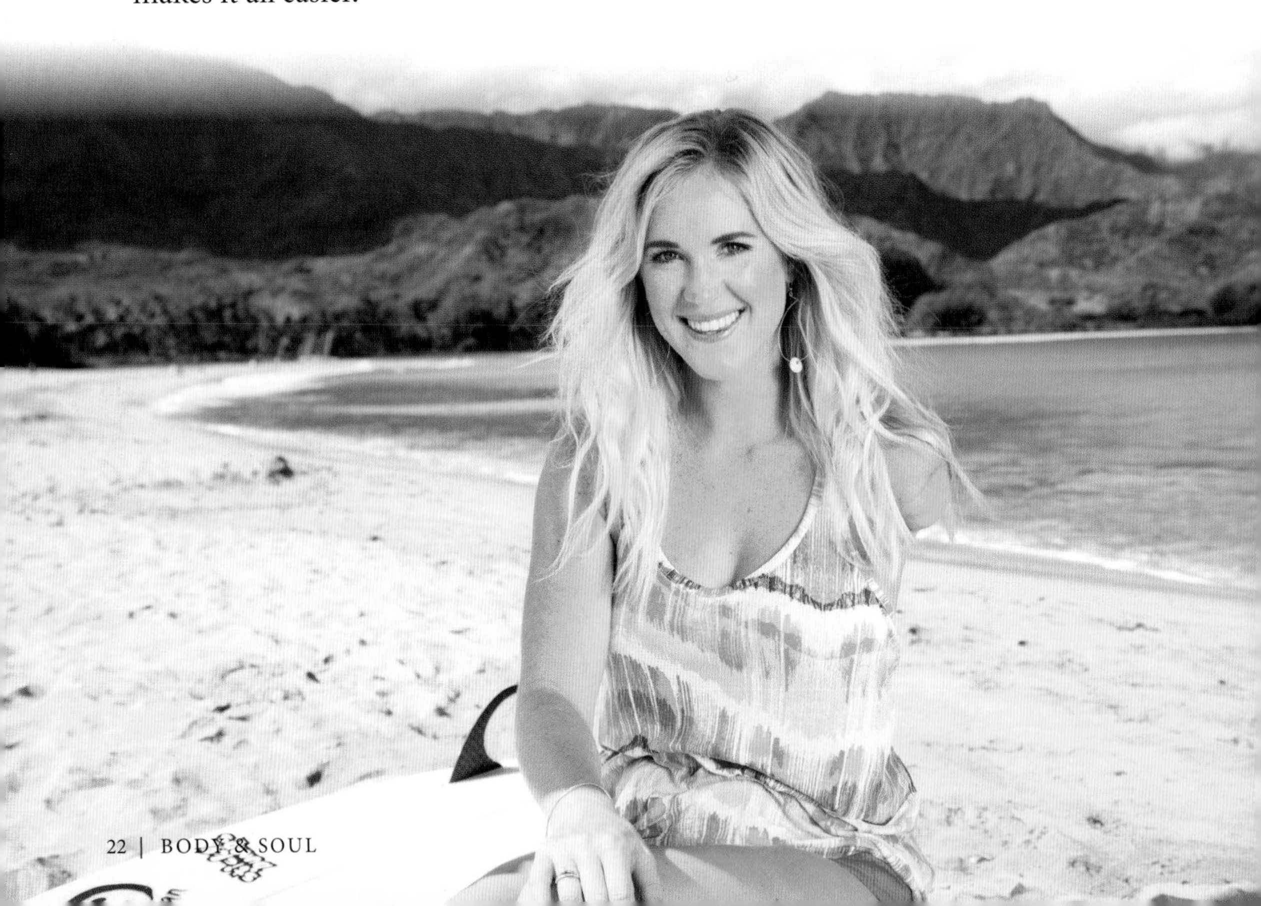

FOUR WAYS TO TREAT YOUR BODY—AND MIND—RIGHT

In need of a little motivation?
Here's how I stay up on down days.

* **Stay positive.**

  No matter how rough the situation is, try to look at the good and stay positive. Sometimes, it's OK to cry and let it out but then try to find something in your life to be thankful for.

* **Feed your body right.**

  I love chocolate, but I have to eat it in moderation otherwise I'll get addicted. Be aware of what you put in your body and experiment with new, healthy bites. You can't say you don't like something until you try it!

* **Break a sweat for God.**

  I really do believe he wants us to take care of our body. I'm not saying you can't go out and have ice cream, but our bodies are created to move and not sit around all day. So get going, find a new, fun, active, hobby.

* **Resist temptation.**

  Flee from temptation, whatever it may be. The great thing is no matter what sin and temptation is trying to get a stronghold in your life, God always provides a way out (1 Corinthians 10:13). And through him, we have the strength to overcome whatever it is.

GO WITH THE PLAN

Like I said, God has a plan for you—just like he does for me. But it's up to you to stick to that plan.

And I'll be the first to admit that's not always easy. Life is full of temptations, whether it's that frosted brownie calling your name or the desire to slack off when you know you should be going for a run.

There are days I want to skip the important things I need to get done and just play in the ocean. But being obedient to God's plan for your life also means overcoming the temptation to ignore him or not follow through with sharing the gospel when you feel a little nudge.

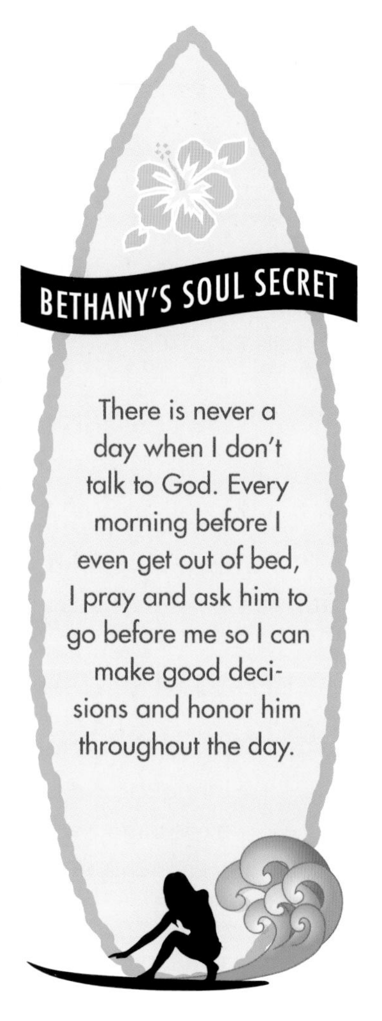

During those tough—and tempting—times, I ask God to guide me to make the best decisions. Just like how I communicate with my best friend, I have to be open, honest, respectful, and upfront with God in order to keep our relationship strong.

Every morning, I pray for guidance to live the healthiest day possible. I pray for motivation to make wise choices. I pray for a positive mindset to be thankful and happy. And I pray for trust and faith to follow the Lord through obstacles and trials. I say something like this:

God, thank you for loving me.

Thank you for blessing me with another wonderful day.

I ask you to be with me and my family and friends today.

Guide me to make wise decisions, bless me with a deeper faith to know you and grow in my love for you, and let me shine your love to others to honor you. I love you! Amen.

One of my favorite Bible verses is Colossians 3:23, "Whatever you do, work at it with all your heart, as working for the Lord." For me, this applies to so many things I face daily, whether it's something awesome like surfing or something I *have* to do like cleaning my house.

Yeah, I may not feel like doing the piles of dishes that have stacked up in my sink, but if I think, "I'm doing it for the Lord," I get the motivation to charge at 'em. Little things build your character, so when something bigger comes your way, you'll feel like you can handle it.

In a world where people make mistakes and let us down, Christ is always there, loving us and wanting us to live for him. And I do—every time I hop up on a surfboard, hit the gym, or down a healthy smoothie, I'm strengthening my faith and my unconditional love for God.

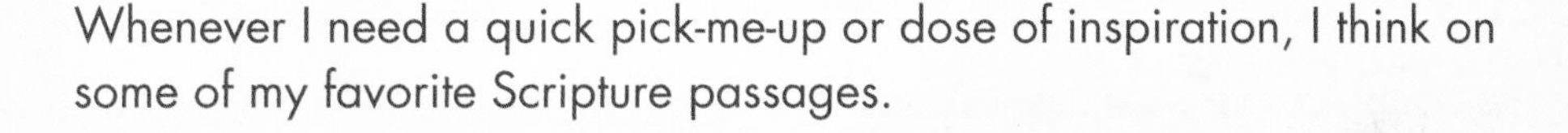

POSITIVE VERSES THAT INSPIRE ME

Whenever I need a quick pick-me-up or dose of inspiration, I think on some of my favorite Scripture passages.

> "Finally, brothers and sisters, whatever is true, whatever is noble, whatever is right, whatever is pure, whatever is lovely, whatever is admirable—if anything is excellent or praiseworthy—think about such things. Whatever you have learned or received or heard from me, or seen in me—put it into practice. And the God of peace will be with you." (Philippians 4:8-9)

> "Therefore, I urge you, brothers and sisters, in view of God's mercy, to offer your bodies as a living sacrifice, holy and pleasing to God—this is your true and proper worship." (Romans 12:1)

> "For I know the plans I have for you," declares the Lord, "plans to prosper you and not to harm you, plans to give you hope and a future." (Jeremiah 29:11)

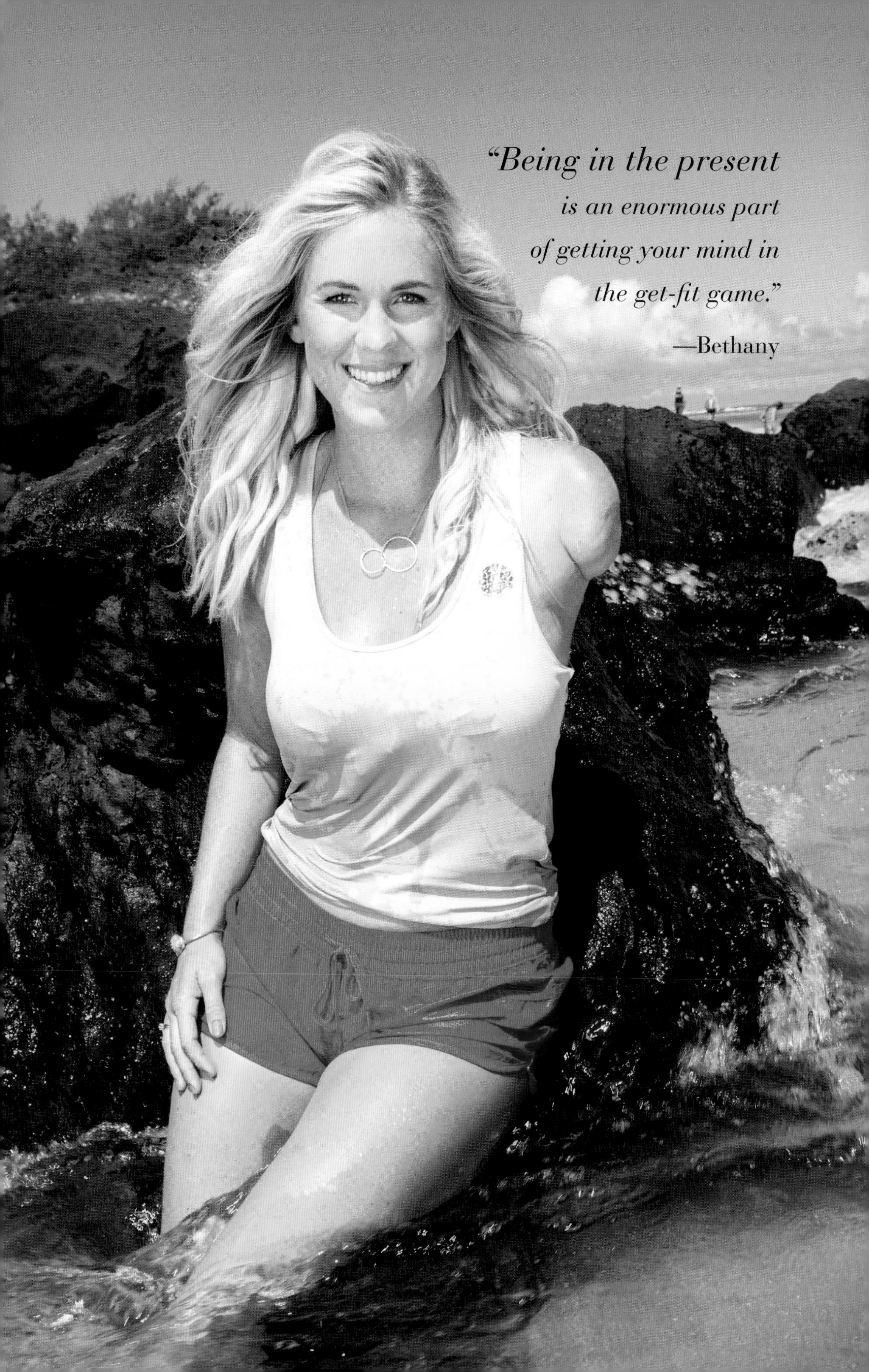
*"Being in the present
is an enormous part
of getting your mind in
the get-fit game."*
—Bethany

CHAPTER 3

Have an Amazing Outlook

(And Let Your Joy Shine)

Here's a big secret to getting in shape and rocking everything you attempt: it's mostly about the right state of mind. Staying positive and having an optimistic outlook can have an enormous influence on every area of your life. If you're consistently negative or doubting your ability, you're less likely to find success in whatever you're going for, whether it's an athletic pursuit or getting good grades in school.

FLIP YOUR MINDSET

A little while back, I was thrown into some tough surfing competitions and went into them feeling discouraged from the start. I didn't perform well or have any fun—it was really frustrating.

Right after that stretch, I started to think about my strengths and look back to the times I was successful. I visualized myself doing my best and didn't let those bad days cross my mind. You know what? The next time I hit the water, I ended up loving the waves, having a blast, and surfing really well.

Every challenge, whether it's a grueling workout or a big competition, is a chance to dig deep and pour your heart out. You won't win them all (and, spoiler, you won't always have your best day at the gym, either) but giving it your all and going for your dreams will make you feel fantastic and build your confidence in the long run. I'm proof that if you have faith and avoid the urge to quit, your life will start to feel even more amazing.

It might seem hard to eat healthy foods all the time or to push your workouts to the next level, but once you flip your mindset to an optimistic one, incredible things will start happening all around you. And guess what? Your taste buds even start to crave your favorite healthy foods! So what are a few of the tricks that help me stay happy, healthy, and super positive? I'll tell ya.

Instead of thinking about all the foods you "shouldn't" eat, consider the astonishing amount of healthy foods God has put on the planet. There are juicy peaches and sweet mangoes, crispy greens that can be tossed in a salad or whipped up into a smoothie, and sweet-yet-refreshing coconut water to be chugged as a post-sweat session treat. When you think like that, focusing on the amazing bounty we're blessed with, you won't even miss greasy potato chips and super sugary cookies.

On the flip side, if your mind is spinning out of control about how yummy cupcakes look and how you wish you could have one but you (ugh!) can't ... but it would be awesome if you could, well, you'll make yourself nuts and all you're thinking about is some pastry and frosting. It's a waste of your time.

The way I see it, some foods give you life (like vegetables and healthy proteins and fruits), and some take it away (like energy-zapping fried and fast foods). Why slow yourself down?

Most of the time, I'm happy to eat clean. I love fruit, and my green smoothies give me such a huge boost in the morning. But I occasionally treat myself to some dark chocolate—yum.

Gluten-free muffins are another indulgence of mine (check out the recipes starting on page 104). The version I whip up is so much better for you than the ones you buy from the store. Plus, who doesn't love baking? And they are fun to share!

I don't feel guilty about eating muffins and chocolate. I just savor each bite and then go back to the clean eating. I know making the best decisions for my body most of the time means I'll feel my best and my performance will be at its peak.

Over time, eating healthy becomes the simplest decision in the world. I don't even think about whether I should have a burger or grilled fish at a barbecue. For me, it's obvious that the fish is the better choice—and the one I'll make just about every time.

Changing my diet has helped me become a better surfer and made my endurance go through the roof. My nutrition trainer, Kirby, helped me with healthy recipes and healthy snacks to munch on the fly.

When I'm eating well, I feel more confident. Eating clean really gives me energy—and not that fake boost sugar might give you, where you crash right down after a short high. Foods should nourish your body and fill you. To eat healthy you don't have to diet or obsess: you simply have to get in the habit of making the best choices for your body, and the transformation will start to occur.

Having an awesome outlook is not just critical for eating right. Looking on the sunny side and thinking about how great you feel when you treat your body with love and respect can help motivate you when you're considering skipping a workout.

Finding it hard to stick to fresh 'n' fab foods? Try keeping a food journal.

When you document what you ate, when you ate, and how you felt before and after, over just a couple of weeks, patterns will start to appear. You'll notice if you're eating late at night out of boredom, if pizza and soda lead to consistent belly aches, or if (surprise!) you feel more energized when you're eating healthy and drinking lots of water.

KIRBY SAYS

Plus—thanks to the endorphins released when you exercise—working out actually boosts your mood. While push-ups might seem like punishment, being active actually zaps stress and can greatly reduce depression. It's proven to lift your spirits and sharpen your mind. And those are just the mental benefits!

Of course, a good sweat sesh will also blast fat from your body, tone your muscles, and ensure you sleep better at night. And it's so fun! Trust me, even if you don't feel that way now, after following my plan for a few weeks, your body and mind will look forward to your daily workouts.

Another way to stay positive and accountable for the goals you're working toward is to surround yourself with uplifting people. It totally helps to have people on the same page as you, who are working toward similar goals and have similar values. When it comes time to throw a sleepover, they'll be the ones psyched to try new recipes and skip the junk food.

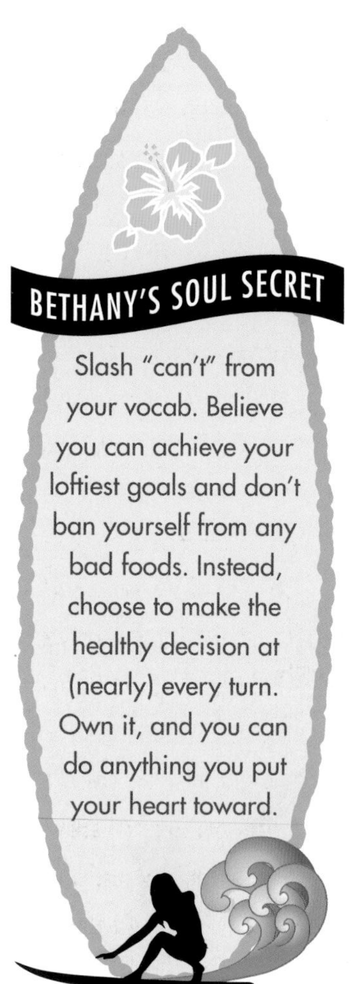

My girlfriends are great about that. We will meet up at the park to work out together, or we'll all go swimming in the ocean.

Recently, a friend wanted to get in better shape, so we decided to go to the gym together regularly. We didn't even do the same exercises, but being there together pushed both of us. We both knew we were being supported. Same thing with my BFF-turned-hubby, Adam: we try new foods together, and if one of us is lacking motivation, the other will suggest going out for a run. I couldn't imagine it any other way!

I had one person in my life who was more negative than the rest. I'm not going to dwell on it here, but she just wasn't uplifting. When you're faced with people like that, keep your bigger picture in mind and focus on your goals and how hard you're working. Don't let someone else's negativity drag you down.

Humble yourselves before the Lord, and he will lift you up.

—JAMES 4:10

My mom and I will go swimming sometimes—we love being in the water together. While some parents are great role models for health, others struggle in this area.

Parents want the best for their kids, but no one is perfect. And some parents haven't (yet) been equipped with the knowledge of healthy living or experienced it themselves. They may feel overwhelmed by circumstances or the busyness of life.

So instead of loading up on fresh foods at the grocery store, they bring home takeout or pull the minivan into McDonald's for dinner. Exercise? It's not a priority, and they might say they don't have time.

It can be hugely challenging to get fit in a household that doesn't value exercise and eating right, but it's not impossible. You can even suggest getting fit as a family.

Offer to pitch in with the cooking (your parents will totally love this!). Ask if you can put a couple new, better-for-you foods on the grocery list each week. Flex that willpower when confronted with a cupboard full of packaged snacks. You can become a wellness inspiration for your entire family. Remember, the Bible says God calls each of us to live a life that's different—and he promises blessings.

Kirby and I believe in the power of mind over matter. No one is forcing you to eat a cookie or to order a super-sized soda or fries, so don't allow yourself to consume them. It will be daunting at first, but making great decisions has a snowball effect: the more good decisions you make, well, the *more* good decisions you'll make.

Every time you reach for water instead of sugary juice or decide to rock a Pilates video instead of chilling on the couch, the more likely you are to make the better choice next time. The opposite is true too, so really focus on making awesome-for-you picks, and soon they will practically start to make themselves.

LIGHT YOUR INNER FIRE

Of all the lessons surfing has taught me (and there are tons), one of the biggest is how it's super important to have something you're passionate about. Along with the grace of God, having something to fight for helped me find happiness and success after my attack.

I could've easily quit surfing and started living a new life, but I knew I loved it too much to just stop. God has given me this passion and ability to ride waves—to be out there and work hard but also have fun with it. I believe he had plans for my life, and he gave me that strength and determination to get back to surfing.

> *For you make me glad by your deeds, Lord; I sing for joy at what your hands have done.*
> —PSALM 92:4

But that's me. You don't need a life-altering event to help you discover your passion and motivation. Lighting your inner fire will make sticking with your plan and achieving your dreams a lot easier. Starting with small dreams and goals now will help you learn how to achieve big dreams as you get older.

Without passion, it's hard to stay committed to a plan and push through the tough days (trust me, they exist). If you're just coasting, unsure about what you're doing, getting up for early a.m. workouts will seem like a chore—and sticking to clean eats will feel impossible.

But once you find something you love, all the effort starts to make sense, and it doesn't seem quite as tough. As the good starts to really show, the challenges feel that much more worth it!

For me, surfing is what gets me stoked, and it motivates me in so many other areas of my life. My love of chasing waves makes it easy to get through difficult workouts, train regularly, and eat clean.

Surfing requires my entire body to be in top shape, which means I'm at the gym doing hard workouts two to three days a week, running two to three days a week, and then doing a fun workout on the other day. (So yeah, I'm working out every day. It's my choice, but I really like it! And, yep, I do have rest days here and there.)

Tons of girls never find their passion for exercise. They might say they want to get in better shape, and then they spend a couple weeks going to the gym and walking on the treadmill or half-heartedly pedaling on the recumbent bike (hint: they're usually the ones texting while they're at it). Has this been you?

BETHANY'S SOUL SECRET

Get some fun, upbeat music going and just rock it! And be sure to do each move properly so you don't get hurt and grow beautiful, strong, confident and great posture you! Don't be afraid to sweat and always push yourself!

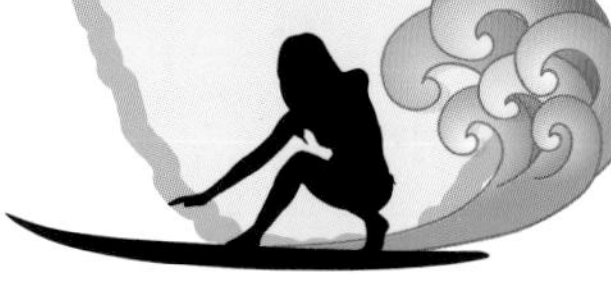

One reason some girls may wonder why they can't stick to a workout routine is because there's no excitement or real motivation. It feels repetitive and boring. Maybe this was you in the past, but it doesn't have to be you in the future.

Why? Because I'm about to help you reach deep into your soul and figure out what you really, truly love in this world. Then I'll share secrets about how to set goals and stay motivated, even on days when working out is the last thing you want to do.

FIND WHAT FIRES YOU UP

Quick, without over-thinking, write down ten healthy things you love to do. It can be making delicious kale salads or jumping rope or doing Pilates or anything else. When you're feeling unmotivated or unsure of your passion, flip back to this list. It's likely to be a gold mine of goodness. And as you find more things you love to do, you can add to the list!

Write down ten things you love to do.

1. ....
2. ....
3. ....
4. ....
5. ....
6. ....
7. ....
8. ....
9. ....
10. ....

If you're having trouble committing to a routine or sticking with your plan, it's time to reevaluate what's on your list. Maybe you wrote down that you love dancing, but if you never want to go to class and can't remember the last time you enjoyed your time in the studio, perhaps it's time to search for a new passion.

Consider this: What really makes you laugh and smile? What activities do you return to, with total ease? If nothing on your list is active, flip to page 84, where I have a list of workouts that are so fun, you'll forget you're exercising. And then commit to doing my trainer Dustin's workouts three times a week. After a while, your body and soul will crave the movement. I promise.

BECOME A GOAL-SETTER

Once you've found what you love, it's time to set goals to hold yourself accountable. I always say, "Having a goal drives you; otherwise, you're just walking aimlessly." Creating a mission for yourself will give you focus and make your efforts more purposeful.

Dustin, Kirby, and I are all fans of setting S.M.A.R.T. goals, which stands for Specific, Measurable, Attainable, Relevant, and Timely. When you create S.M.A.R.T. goals, you're really setting yourself up for success. Simply aiming to "get in shape" is vague, which is why so many people fall off their path. Instead, try setting a goal like this:

* Shave thirty seconds off my mile time within two months so I can meet the standards the JV soccer coach has set.
* Start doing Pilates videos at home to improve my core for the upcoming swim season.
* In addition to cardio, go to yoga or have a good stretch sesh twice a week until November, to up my flexibility for cheerleading.

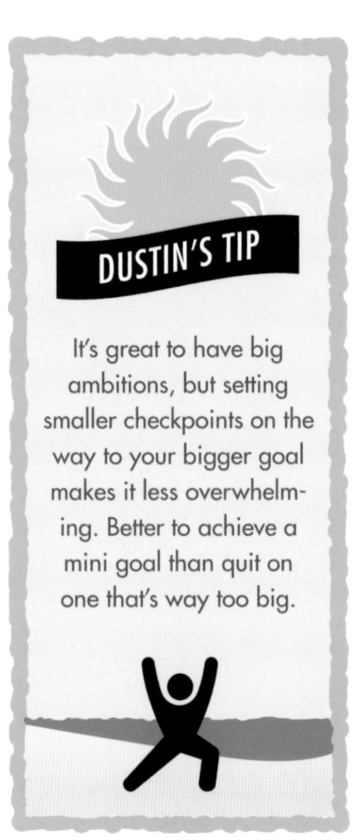

As driven as I am and as you might be, no one is going to achieve all her goals, all of the time. When I fall short, I take time to reevaluate my target and see if it was realistic for me. If it wasn't, I'll reset it and get back to action. Then, if I still need more motivation, I'll ask a friend or trainer to help me out. You could do the same, or even sign up for a class to help hone your skills.

STAY PRESENT

Here's something you should know about surfing: when you're about to pop up on your board, your entire body is focused on one thing—catch the wave that's coming your way.

Your brain is so busy telling your body what to do—paddle faster, find your balance—there's not a second to focus about the inconsequential things in life. I'm not worried about how I look in my suit or if my ponytail is out of place. Out in the water, it's just about me and God and the waves. It's perfect.

Being in the present is an enormous part of getting your mind in the get-fit game. When your mind drifts, you're inevitably going to get distracted or start thinking about how tough the task at hand is.

Picture this: You're out sprinting on the track. You're halfway through an intense workout, and you're getting tired. You could start obsessing about all the work ahead of you, whining to yourself about how darn hard this is.

Or you could concentrate on the immediate: *I'm getting a drink of water and am grateful for the hydration. My thighs might hurt, but my breathing is really great. I'm taking a quick stretch break. I'm getting back to my running and am happy God gave me the ability to run.*

Getting in shape and honing your abilities in any area of your life requires repetition. I've paddled out to countless waves, done a zillion squats, run tons of miles, and sipped gallons of coconut water. I could get bored with it, but I know all the hours I spend in the gym, on the road, and in the water are what make me feel the best. (See? This is why it's so critical to do something you're passionate about.)

It's also important to search for the joy and pleasure in the things you do all the time. You might not love to run, but that doesn't mean you have to dread each and every endurance-boosting jog. Instead, try to find what you do enjoy about your trots—maybe you're blessed with amazing scenery or you often cruise past a super-cute puppy or you love how you can just let your mind wander as you chug along.

KICK IT UP A NOTCH

I'm really blessed to work with Kirby and Dustin. They're supportive and push me on days when I'm feeling off, and I am always accountable to them.

But at the end of the day, I am the one who has to work hard in the gym, eat clean, and be present for myself and God every single day. It might be easy to look at me and other pro athletes and think, "Oh, I'd sooo be in better shape if I had a coach like she does."

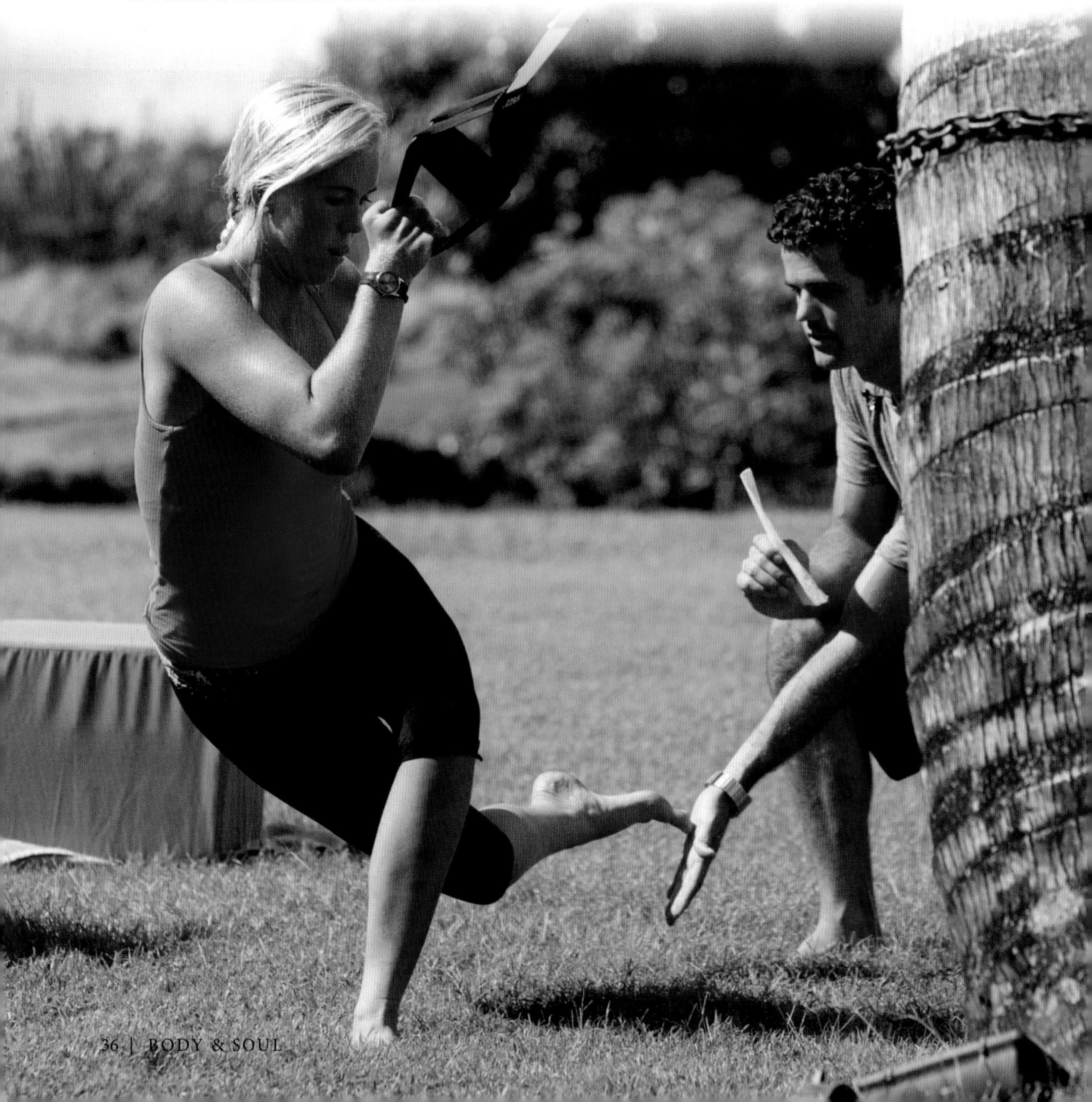

And maybe that's true for some people, but I honestly believe everything it takes to succeed and get a healthy body is within your reach. Yep, everything.

You're the one who has to push yourself on those days when you just want to slack. You're the one who has to turn down Snickers ice cream when you're out with your friends, and they want to indulge yet again. You're the one who has to want it and work for it. Even if you had an amazing coach, he or she couldn't really make you run faster or lift more or try harder. It has to be in your soul. And trust me, it's there.

One way to push yourself is to keep track of your workouts in a notebook or with an app like MapMyRun (check out iTunes for tons of exercise trackers). Seeing how much you've improved over time will give you a huge boost. And if you're plateauing and no longer seeing changes? You can take a look back at what you've been doing, look inside yourself, and see what you can tweak to get even better or work harder.

Of course, you don't want to injure yourself or go to extremes. But many girls don't strive to get faster or stronger, and in the end, their workouts suffer and get boring. We gotta keep it fresh!

That's why having a goal is so important, but also why challenging yourself and checking in is key. Are you adding reps or more weight when you have a strength day? Are you going on long runs when you're doing cardio, or do you take a short cut? Be honest with yourself, and know that no one else can do the work for you.

Sitting at a computer might not get you in great shape, but the Internet can be a huge resource when it comes to finding new workouts and recipes. I'm always posting great tips on my blog, and Dustin and Kirby often update their Facebook pages with new recipes, tips, and all kinds of motivation. Always make sure you're taking health advice from a reliable, certified source. I don't want you to get hurt or follow an unhealthy eating plan.

Being educated on living well can also help if you're surrounded with unsupportive people. They might insist that it's not a big deal if you have another slice of pizza, but knowing why you nourish your body the way you do will help you stay true to your soul.

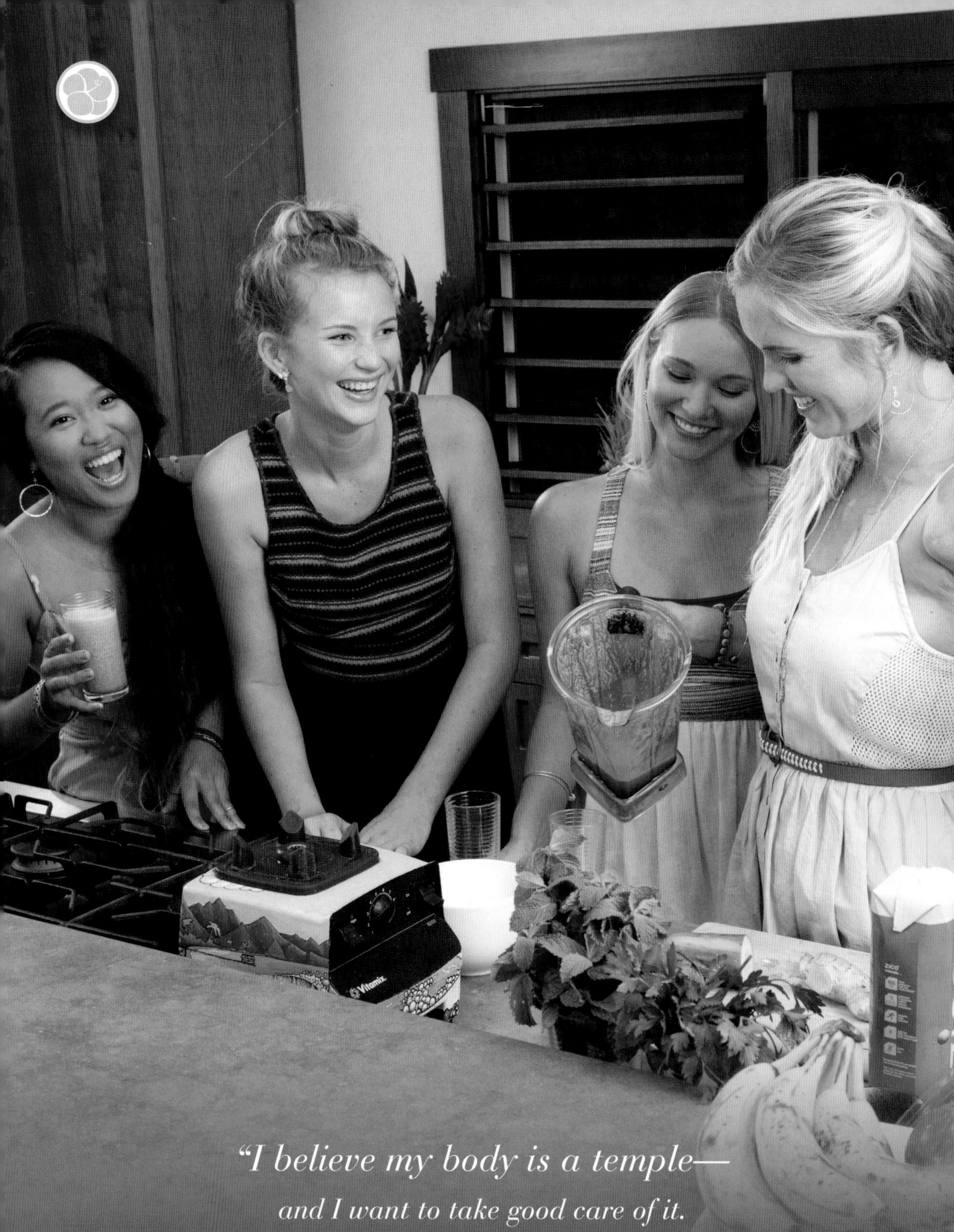

"I believe my body is a temple—
and I want to take good care of it.
It's important for me to make smart choices
and eat foods that give me all the nutrients I need."

–Bethany

CHAPTER 4

Get Your Eat On

As a pro surfer, paying attention to what I eat is essential—I need to stay fueled through all the activities I do throughout the day!

Some people can get away with plowing through tons of junk food and still look like they're in good shape. And some athletes use their major calorie-busting workouts as a kind of nutritional get-out-of-jail-free card—they eat whatever they want, thinking they'll "burn it off" later.

BODY COMPOSITION

But it doesn't exactly work that way. Some girls might look thin, but if they're eating the wrong foods, their insides aren't in tip-top shape. That's because of body composition—a.k.a. what your body is made up of, like fat, bone, and muscle. A healthy composition is one that's greater in healthy tissue and lean muscle, with a low percentage of fat. That comes from exercising, being properly hydrated and fueling your body with good-for-you foods.

On the flip side, an unhealthy composition is one that has a higher fat to muscle ratio due to eating lots of junk and not getting enough exercise. But it's not always possible to see that from the outside. Why is just looking like you are in "good" shape on the outside an issue? Because not taking proper care of your body will catch up with you over time and could lead to major health problems.

Crazy enough, when we exercise, we are working hard to break-down our bodies. This weakness is just temporary—our bodies respond by building muscle and getting stronger (see, you knew an upside was coming!). The rate at which we can recover from our workouts is in direct relation to how healthy we hydrate and eat.

Friends say to me all the time, "If I work out really hard it's OK to have a splurge, right?" But what you eat post-workout affects how your body can repair itself ... that's why it's critical to get in tons of nutrients and water. If you're refueling with Twizzlers, your body isn't getting the critical building blocks it needs to gain that strength back.

I don't take the work hard/splurge hard approach to eating. I believe my body is a temple—and I want to take good care of it. It's important for me to make smart choices and eat foods that give me all the nutrients I need. Sure, I want to be confident in my bikini when I'm at the beach or surfing, but (even more important) I want my insides really healthy, too

So what is important to understand is that just because you are "skinny" or appear healthy doesn't mean you can live unhealthy without future consequences.

Knowing why you are doing something makes it easier to stay committed.

Kale might not be your favorite, but understanding that it gives your body vital nutrients might prompt you to incorporate it in your dinner. Even if you don't love posture work, it's vital to keep your balance top-notch. Keeping your body standing tall with good poise will help keep you injury-free. This knowlege can be a big motivator.

KIRBY SAYS

WHAT MAKES A GOOD PROTEIN?

Protein is found in everything from nuts and beans to animal products. But not all proteins are created equal. A fast-food hamburger, for example, might be loaded up with salt and made from beef that comes from cows hopped up on antibiotics (which promote growth in animals, but are not great for humans). A cage-free organic egg, on the other hand, is a great source of protein.

When you're on the hunt for protein, look for words like organic, cage-free, antibiotic-free, hormone-free, nitrate-free, grass-fed, local free-range, and sustainable to ensure you're getting the purest meat, milk, fish, and eggs around.

Keep in mind, too, that multiple sources for macronutrients (i.e. protien, fats, carbs) are ideal. Don't rely only on one type. There are many fods that have protein, aside from meats and dairy products: nuts, seeds, beans, quinoa, and even some veggies and greens such as kale. See portion chart on page 47.

THE MYTH ABOUT CARBS

As I mentioned a little while back, carbohydrates are quite literally a key to life. So why do so many people get crazy about cutting carbs?

It's best to think about carbs going across a spectrum: some are void of vitamins and minerals and packed with sugar, and some are rich in fiber and loaded with nutrients, which means they're slower to digest.

A longer digestion period means your blood sugar stays even, instead of spiking up (like after eating candy). Eating nutritious foods at regular intervals helps balance your metabolism, which is how your body uses the energy it's given.

A handy way to consider which carbs are good and which are less-than-fab is the Glycemic Index (GI), which gives foods a number based on how slowly or quickly they cause your blood sugar to rise.

Carbs with a high GI release glucose (that's sugar) quickly—think pretzels, white bread, white rice, and breakfast cereals. Those with a low GI have fiber, which keeps you feeling full longer. This group includes lots of fruits and vegetables, whole grains, and seeds. This probably won't shock you to read: foods with a low GI are better for you.

You will notice that my go-to foods in this category are vegetables and fruits. These are the highest in nutritional value. As far as grains go, I like quinoa, and wild and brown rice.

DON'T FEAR FATS

There are tons of fad diets out there, but one trend that has stuck around for ages is America's obsession with low-fat foods. As Kirby always says, fat doesn't make you fat.

On the contrary, good fats (like the ones found in macadamia nuts, olive oil, coconut oil, and avocados) can help give you energy, aid in digestion, and keep your heart healthy. Along with proteins, fats keep hunger pangs at bay, which means you'll feel fuller longer.

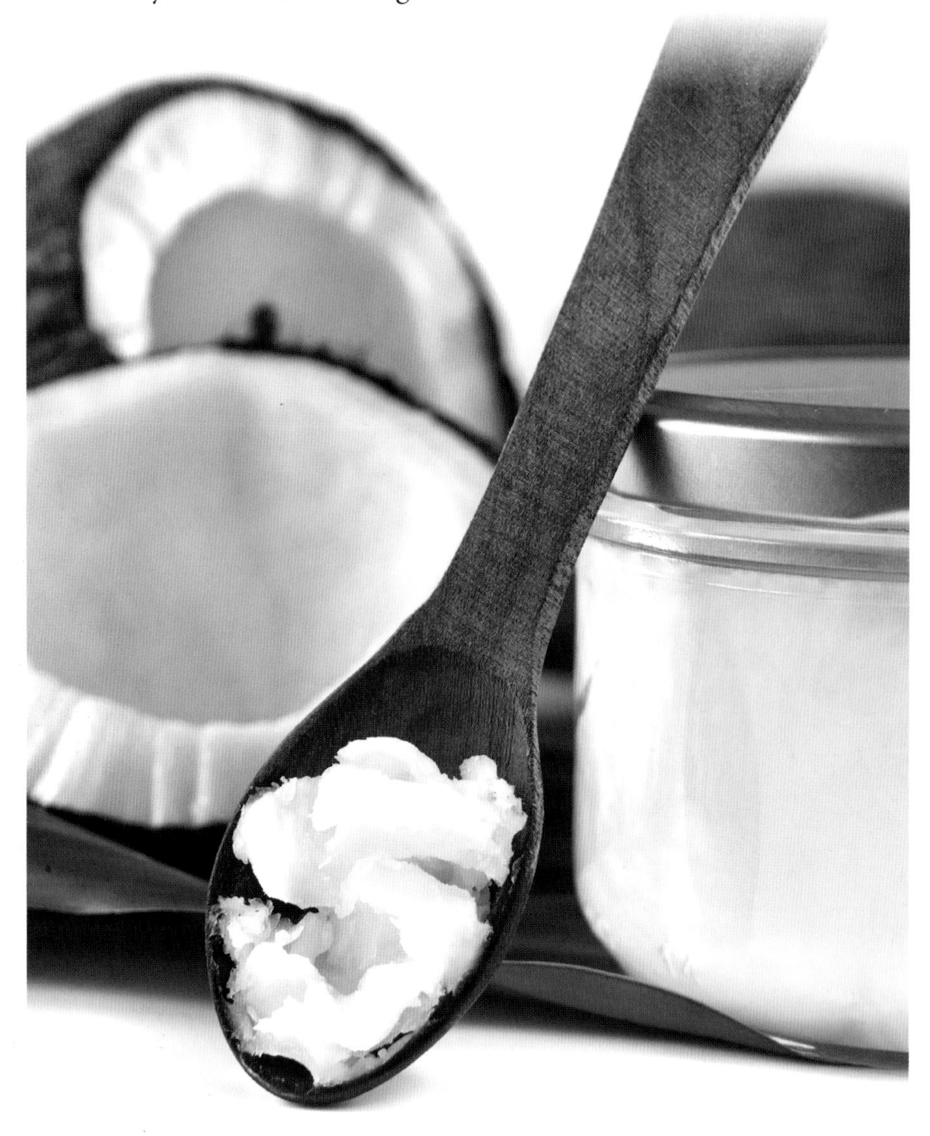

But be on guard when a label says "low fat." Often that means the food has been processed to have less fat but more sugar. And seriously avoid "trans fats," also known as "partially hydrogenated oils." Trans fats are associated with all sorts of problems like high cholesterol and strokes.

Now that you know the basics, here are seven more secrets that will help you make the best decisions for your body.

SMART EATING SECRET #1

GET INFORMED

As you grow and change, it's important to know how your body is affected by what you eat and drink.

Here's a crash course in nutrition (don't worry, it won't be long). First, there are macronutrients—proteins, fats, and carbohydrates.

Basically, macronutrients make up the majority of our diet, and they are vital for energy, cell growth and repair, and, well, living. Fats and proteins can be found in meats, beans, and milk, and carbohydrates can be found in everything from potatoes to cookies.

Then there are micronutrients. Micronutrients are basically vitamins and minerals, and they're different from macronutrients because they are only needed in very small amounts, but they are still essential for good health. Micronutrients help with critical functions in your body—which is why eating a balanced and varied diet is so critical. Why can this be tricky? Well, eating well is all about getting the right amount of the right nutrients at the right time.

Salt, for example, is a mineral that's essential for functions in the body. There are two main types of salt: table salt and sea salt. Sea salt is natural and comes from the wonderful sea with electrolytes and trace minerals the way God intended it. Table salt is made in a chemical lab where sodium and chloride are combined to create something that tastes very "salty" but causes problems internally. Too much sodium and you'll start to have heart problems.

Luckily, eating a diet that's full of colorful, fresh foods and plenty of variety can ensure you're getting each and every vitamin and mineral on the list. And put the emphasis on colorful: eating a wide range of hues is one way to ensure you're filling your body with what it needs. And have some sea salt in your pantry for when you need it.

If you try to eat a range of good fats, good proteins, and good carbohydrates (more on those in a sec) and drink plenty of good water, you'll get strong and stay healthy. But when people skip veggies, sip lots of soda, and start slashing entire macronutrients from their diet (like carbs), that's when problems come.

Let's say you're low on vitamin B12, which is found in dairy, eggs, meat, and fish. That one tiny vitamin deficiency can lead to depression, fatigue, and nerve damage. And that's just one vitamin—there are thirteen total which are essential for humans. Toss in other minerals (like calcium and iron), which are necessary for everything from bone health to immunity, and deciding what to have for lunch takes on a whole new meaning.

To figure out how much to eat at a meal, check out our recipes in Chapter eight and the portion chart on page 47. Get used to really listening to your body.

SMART EATING SECRET #2

EAT CLOSE TO THE SOURCE

Trust me, I like technology as much as the next girl. I'm constantly texting with my friends, and writing my blog means I can keep in touch with all of you girls. But one area of our lives where more technology isn't always better is in the kitchen.

Scientists have figured out how to make massive amounts of low-fat foods and foods that last on the shelves for ages. (I'm looking at you, Twinkies.) It really amazes me to see all the junk that's in the grocery store posing as healthy eats but are really filled with salt, sugar, and chemicals. Ick. The bottom line? No matter what the label says, nothing beats good ol' vegetables and fruits for true nourishment.

I feed my body as many local, organic, and natural foods as possible. It's the easiest way to ensure what you're putting in your body is fresh, loaded with energy, and good for you.

As Kirby puts it, "whole food is good food." It's the food God has given us, and you can find it in the sea, in the ground, and on trees all around you. It's always best to eat foods closest to their natural form, when they contain the most nutrients. That means before the food has been processed with added fats, sugars, and chemicals and then put into a package. Try to eat local, organic fruits, vegetables, and proteins. Not only is this healthier, but you are eating foods closer to their source (and supporting your local community at the same time—always a good thing).

For example, spinach is so good for you, and it's really delicious in salads and eggs in the morning. Spinach gets less healthy, however, when it's whipped up into a chemical-and salt-laden dip in a factory, placed in a jar, and sent out to your supermarket.

The same thing is true for apples when they get made into those little pies sold in convenience stores. Or a tomato that's been made into sauce and plunked onto a frozen pizza. At one point, each of those fruits and veggies was a whole food, but once it's processed, the nutritional benefits are zapped.

I can't stress enough how vital it is to cut processed foods out of your diet. Kirby always says to me, "If you want to be healthy, you have to do healthy things."

Avoiding processed foods is one huge step you can take on your journey to a healthier lifestyle. Sure, avoiding processed foods can be a challenge. After all, our world is filled with packaged, frozen, canned, and fast foods—not to mention convenience. But the additives and unhealthy trans fats found in a lot of these foods have been linked to everything from depression to obesity.

Even in healthy grocery stores, there are aisles and aisles of "natural" cookies and frozen dinners. And sure, they may be less processed and healthier than their regular counterparts, but the truth is, making your own food is always best. Plus, it's so much fun!

SMART EATING SECRET #3

KEEP IT FRESH AND FUN

Opting to eat only the foods created by God can seem overwhelming, but there's really an endless supply of foods available.

Each season, God gives us a fresh bounty to choose from, and it's different all over the country. In Hawaii, summer months mean melons and mangoes. Fall gives us sweet tangerines and a huge bounty of bananas, while avocados are available through winter. Pineapples and fish come to us fresh at all times of the year—we're so blessed.

Then God said, "I give you every seed-bearing plant on the face of the whole earth and every tree that has fruit with seed in it. They will be yours for food."

—GENESIS 1:29

Getting to know the rhythm of the seasons and what grows in your area at different times will help you shake up what you put on your plate and keep your palate guessing.

One way I track what's freshest is by going to my local farmer's market. Check your newspaper or go online to find a farmer's market near you. They have way more than just vegetables too. You can often find pretty gifts, fresh-cut flowers, and locally-made soaps. Farmer's markets are so much fun! Especially with friends. I love checking out different farmer's markets when I travel.

SMART EATING SECRET #4

GET SMART

Even at farmer's markets and natural food stores—places designed to sell the healthiest foods on God's green earth—you'll find not-so-great choices.

At farmer's markets, there are potatoes being fried into chips, popcorn doused in sugar and oil, and more baked goods than you can even imagine.

The same is true in grocery stores. Even at the ones that say they're filled with natural, whole, and healthy foods, you need to check the labels to avoid bad-for-you foods wrapped up in a deceivingly healthy-looking package. (Discouraging, I know).

Kirby says the best way to avoid bad stuff in the store is to shop around the perimeter of the place. That's where the freshest, healthiest foods are, every time. It's where the fish sits on ice, where the butcher is carving meat, and where fresh apples are available by the pound.

Start in the massive area dedicated to fruits and vegetables, and be mindful as you pick out your pears, clementines, and arugula.

Then, move on to the meats, looking for organic, hormone-free chicken before heading to the seafood counter for sustainable fish. You might need to duck into the interior section for brown rice or coconut milk, but for the most part, it's all about the fresh options.

Be especially careful when you reach the checkout. That's where the clever people who run stores often load up the junk food for "impulse purchases." You'll find a sea of chips, soda, and more candy than you can imagine—skip it all.

SMART EATING SECRET #5

PORTION LIKE A PRO

It's no secret we live in a super-sized world. Food portions in restaurants have increased over the years, and so have people's waistlines. But you don't have to fall victim to portion distortion.

When you go out to eat with your friends or family, ask for a half portion or go splitsies on an entree. Another idea is to just order an appetizer—which often is big enough to be a meal on its own.

Portions at home can be just as confusing, especially if your parents insist you finish everything on your plate or bring home giant bagels, brownies, and bags of chips.

Hand Symbol	Food Focus	Best Choices (Our Faves)
	VEGGIES: should be more than your hand size and be included with every meal.	Organic and local spinach, kale, broccoli, bell peppers, mushrooms, carrots, cauliflower, zucchini, onion, butternut squash, beets. (This list could go on and on, veggies are amazing!)
	HIGH QUALITY FATS & OILS: up to 2 tbsps. per serving.	Coconut oil, olive oil (best used uncooked), macadamia nut oil, avocado oil and avocado, sesame oil, almond butter, sunflower seed butter.
	MEATS: size and thickness of palm.	Fresh non-farmed fish, organic free-range non-grain fed chicken, grass fed organic beef, organic grass fed lamb, organic free-range eggs.
	FRUIT: size and thickness of palm.	Applies, blueberries, raspberry, pineapple, lemon, peaches, avocado, banana.
	STARCHES: size and thickness of palm.	Quinoa, wild rice, brown rice, sweet potato, pinto beans, black beans, lentils.
	NUTS & SEEDS: and snacks other than veggies.	Raw nuts (almonds, cashews, macadamia nuts, walnuts, pecans), seeds (sunflower, pumpkin), organic popcorn, rice chips, dried fruit.

SMART EATING SECRET #6

MAKE MEALTIME SACRED

How you eat is just as important as what you eat. So many of us are constantly on the go, so lots of girls eat meals on the bus, rushed between classes, or alone in front of the television. One way to slow down your eating and enjoy your food is to make mealtime intentional.

My meals always have a nice rhythm to them: I prepare everything, pray, and then eat, making sure to savor every bite. It's always best to eat in a relaxed, thankful way. Chew your food well and eat slowly so you'll know when you are full. I often eat too fast and I'm trying to work on this!

When you're eating mindfully, you're more likely to stop eating when you're full. Instead, you'll be able to appreciate God's work as you slowly nourish and replenish your body.

SMART EATING SECRET #7

TIMING IS EVERYTHING

I always eat within thirty minutes of waking up, which ensures I don't get too hungry before breakfast. Then I try to eat every three hours, and I always stop eating at least ninety minutes before bedtime. Sticking with a rigid schedule will help ensure you don't eat out of boredom, nervousness, or any other emotion.

Often when girls try to "eat healthier," they actually go on scary diets, which leave them tired and depleted of nutrients. Some girls will skip meals in order to lose weight, but it totally backfires. If you go too long without eating, your body will get too hungry, and you'll make worse choices.

Kirby recommends eating three meals daily and two to three nutritious snacks in between, which will keep your energy levels up and your blood sugar even. When you skip meals, your body stops burning fuel, so your metabolism comes to a halt—that's why eating frequently is so important—and why it's unhealthy to ditch a meal.

In chapter 8, Kirby has shared plenty of recipes—including meals, smoothies, and yummy desserts—and each one will support your new, healthy ways. Plus, they're so good you'll forget they're good for you!

SMART EATING SECRET #8

MAKE A PLAN

I'm always looking for fresh, yummy eats to help me stay in great shape—and fabulous health—even when I'm traveling or when things are hectic. I don't use being on the road as an excuse to eat tons of fast food or just down whatever's in front of me. With a little planning, I'm able to nosh nourishing foods, no matter how crazy things get.

Being prepared for your day-to-day schedule as best you can ensures you'll stay on track with your goals. As Dustin and Kirby like to say, if you don't make a plan, you plan to fail. You can't wait until the last minute to do things.

During the weekend (when you're less likely to be busy with school or tons of extra-curriculars), grab your family and go food shopping for the week. Then set aside a couple hours to pre-make meals for the next seven days (just make sure to freeze them in air-tight containers). It will take the guesswork out of what to eat every night, plus save you loads of time.

Practically half of my year is spent on the road. If I'm not surfing in a competition or on an adventure surf trip with my sponsor Rip Curl, I might be found somewhere else in the world doing an appearance or a speaking event.

But just because I'm away from the comforts of my home isn't an excuse to get lazy. Dustin always points out that laziness fuels laziness; activity fuels activity. So work out and eat right no matter where you are.

If I'm going on a plane, I always make sure to pack healthy snacks like apples, or another of my favorites—kale chips. Sometimes I'll bring pre-sliced celery or carrots and throw them in a Tupperware with a scoop of almond butter. You can pack smart before going to school or when you have a

Create a meal plan that produces an outcome you desire.

If you want to feel energized and look your best, plan ahead to make sure you're ready at each and every meal and snack time. For me, that means cutting up apples, bringing almond butter along to competitions, and keeping a water bottle handy when I leave the house. A little preparation goes a long way.

KIRBY SAYS

full day of sports, so you won't have to settle for junk food when your fridge or kitchen counter isn't nearby.

Do the same planning when you're eating out. Many restaurants list their menus online, and I always do research on my destinations beforehand. The Yelp app can help your search for healthy hot spots. Type in search terms like "organic restaurant." I'm also never afraid to speak up and ask the server to modify a dish to fit my needs.

So what are some things you can do to switch up your meals out? For starters, send the bread back. Research has shown that if you start your meal with bread, you usually end up eating dessert because it pretty much shuts down the mechanism that tells you when you're full. And when most meals come with starch as a side, like rice or mashed potatoes, ask for raw, sautéed, or even mixed veggies instead.

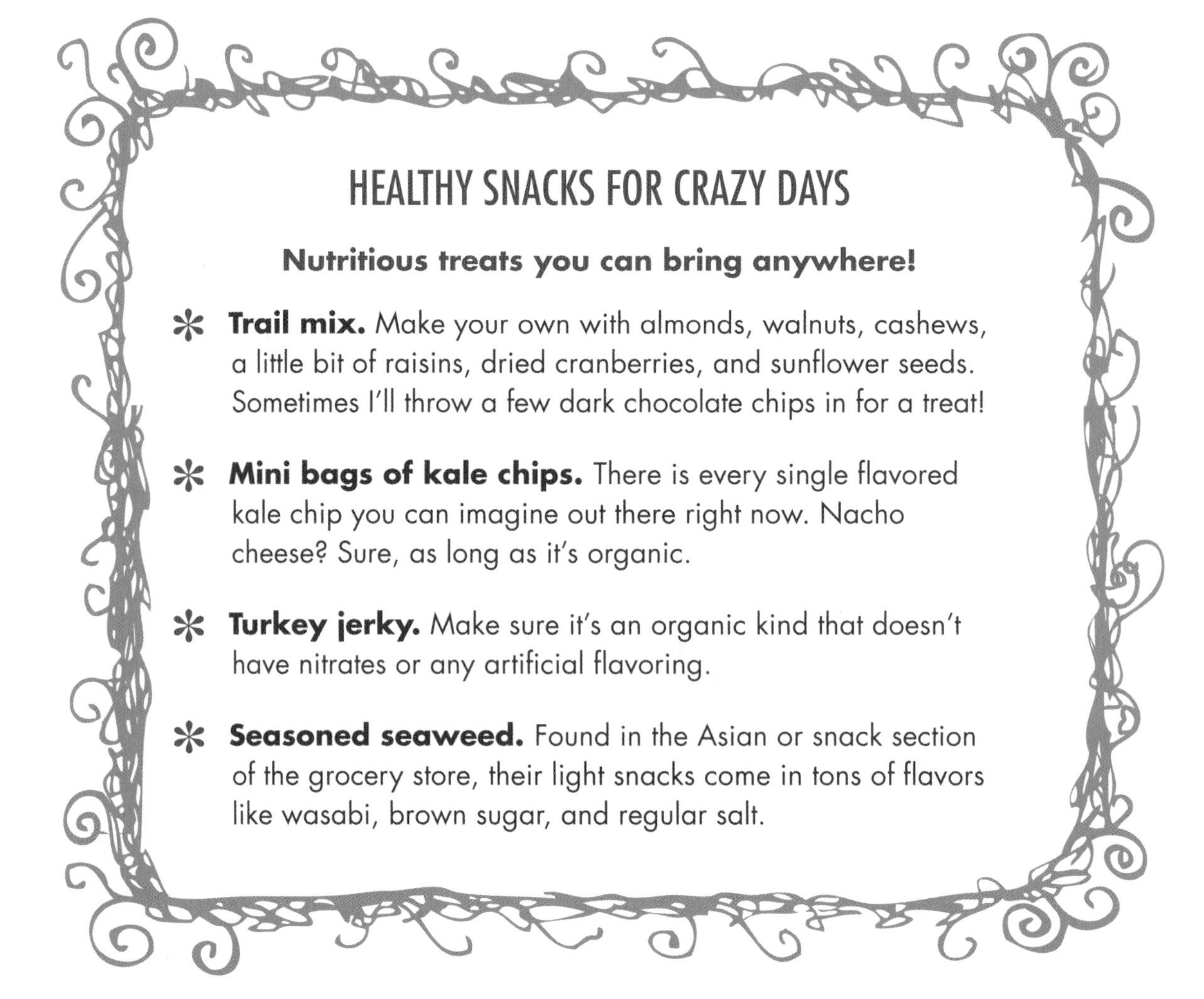

HEALTHY SNACKS FOR CRAZY DAYS

Nutritious treats you can bring anywhere!

* **Trail mix.** Make your own with almonds, walnuts, cashews, a little bit of raisins, dried cranberries, and sunflower seeds. Sometimes I'll throw a few dark chocolate chips in for a treat!
* **Mini bags of kale chips.** There is every single flavored kale chip you can imagine out there right now. Nacho cheese? Sure, as long as it's organic.
* **Turkey jerky.** Make sure it's an organic kind that doesn't have nitrates or any artificial flavoring.
* **Seasoned seaweed.** Found in the Asian or snack section of the grocery store, their light snacks come in tons of flavors like wasabi, brown sugar, and regular salt.

SMART EATING SECRET #9

WHAT YOU DRINK

It's no secret I love the ocean, but my appreciation for water doesn't end at the shore. Downing plenty of water is critical too.

While you've probably heard it before, the importance of filling up on pure, fresh H20 shouldn't be ignored. In fact, drinking more water is the first change you should make to your lifestyle.

Aim to drink at least 8-12 cups each day. Scientific research says there is an equation that will help you drink the appropriate amount of H2O:

YOU (body weight in pounds) divided by 2
= number of ounces of water to drink per day.

I actually drink more like twelve cups each and every day. I keep water at my bedside and drink before I crash, sometimes in the middle of the night, and first thing in the morning. It's become habit for me—and I like the habit!

Staying hydrated is essential to keeping every part of your body functioning at tip-top condition, keeping your energy up, and keeping junk food cravings at bay. (A lot of times when you think you're hungry, your body is actually thirsty.)

As an athlete, I wouldn't be able to get through my toughest competitions and workouts if I was dehydrated—it literally would stop me in my tracks.

Chugging water should be easy enough, but many of us are consistently dehydrated. To avoid the overeating, headaches, and sluggishness that come with dehydration, always carry a water bottle around with you. (Make sure to find one that is free of BPA, a nasty industrial chemical that may be super harmful.)

WATER
Drink it up!

Pure water keeps your body working at its best, making your skin glow, allowing your muscles to power through a workout, and helping icky toxins get flushed out of your system.

KIRBY SAYS

Kirby and I both love the bottles marked with ounces along the side so you can easily figure out exactly how much of the good stuff you've downed. You can also keep four or five hair elastics or rubber bands on your bottle, and pull one off every time you've made your way through.

Is drinking tons of water getting super dull? Instead of skipping this essential practice or drinking a sugary substitute, change it up. Lemon water is my go-to when I want a li'l flavor. If you want to add flavor to your water, toss fruit into your pitcher, add herbs to ice cubes, or try some combo of both. Learn to love water!

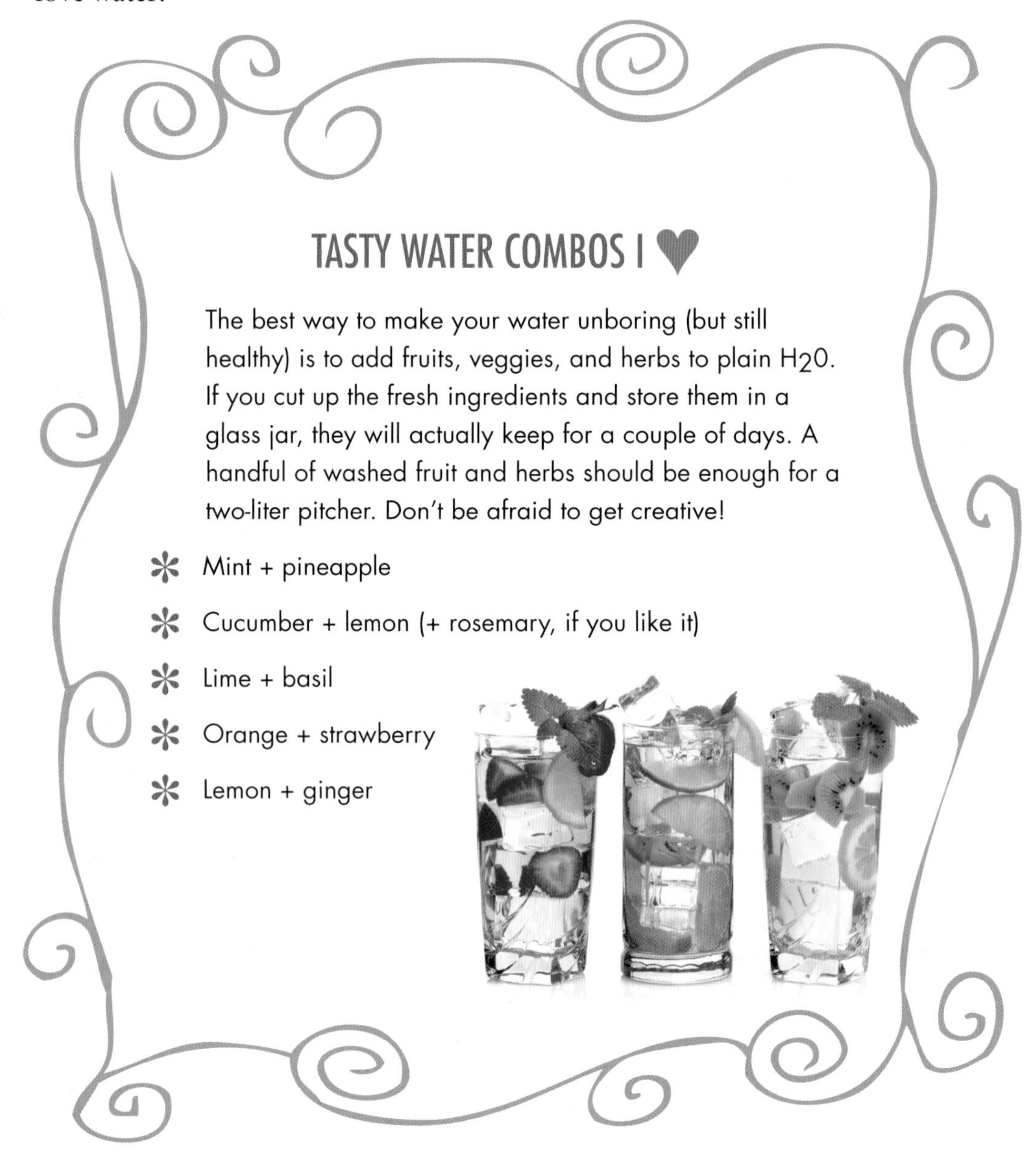

TASTY WATER COMBOS I ♥

The best way to make your water unboring (but still healthy) is to add fruits, veggies, and herbs to plain H_2O. If you cut up the fresh ingredients and store them in a glass jar, they will actually keep for a couple of days. A handful of washed fruit and herbs should be enough for a two-liter pitcher. Don't be afraid to get creative!

- Mint + pineapple
- Cucumber + lemon (+ rosemary, if you like it)
- Lime + basil
- Orange + strawberry
- Lemon + ginger

There are some drinks that seem like they should be healthy but are secretly a nutritional nightmare. "Fake" juices (the ones made from concentrate or high-fructose corn syrup or even worse —artificial sweeteners/colors/flavors), sports drinks, and "waters with vitamins" pop into my head. All of them have been cleverly marketed to seem like the perfect alternative, but they are basically just sugar and water.

Think of any non-water beverage like a snack.

Even juice, which seems healthy (fruit), can be filled with tons of extra sugar. Alternative go-to drinks: water, coconut water, unsweetened, all-natural teas, and sparkling water with a dash of fruit juice (fresh if possible) or a squeeze of citrus (lemon and lime are faves).

KIRBY SAYS

Girls pick up those bottles *thinking* they are about to nourish their bodies, but they are actually just weighing themselves down. How frustrating. Be sure to check labels and skip anything that has sugar, high-fructose corn syrup, or artificial sweeteners, colors, or flavors as the top ingredients.

If you crave juice, treat yourself to a homemade version. This way you know exactly what is in it and ensures you are not consuming something that is processed, flavored, or adds sugars. Every morning, I start my day with a green smoothie. It revs up my body, gives me a burst of vitamins, and gets me ready to take on everything the day is gonna bring, whether that's time on the water, in the gym, or traveling to a big competition. Sure, it might take a little extra time in the morning, but imagine arriving at school feeling healthy, energized, and totally ready for whatever comes your way.

It's an amazing feeling, and I think everyone should kick off the day with this nutrient-filled drink. Even if you think you don't want to sip your greens, just try it. Green smoothies are addictive—and incredibly good for you.

Coconut water is another one of my favorite ways to hydrate—tasty but still healthy. Coconut water is a Hawaiian staple, and now this tropical beverage is easy to find on the mainland, which makes me very happy when I'm traveling.

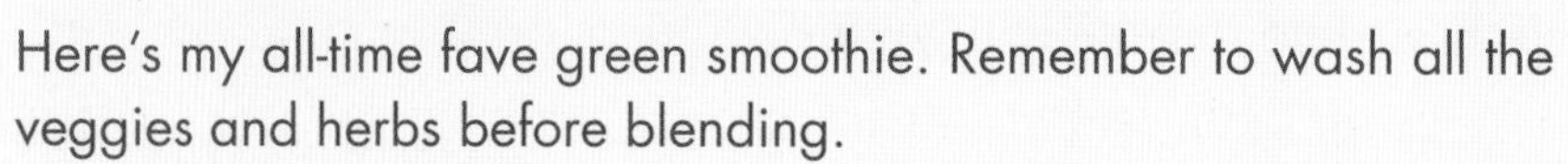

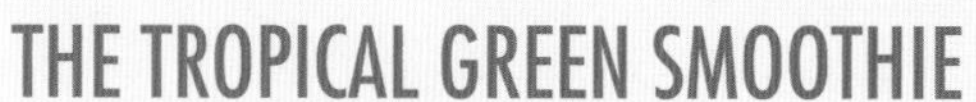

THE TROPICAL GREEN SMOOTHIE

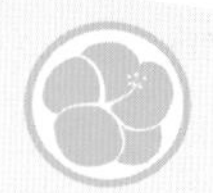

Here's my all-time fave green smoothie. Remember to wash all the veggies and herbs before blending.

- 1 handful spinach or kale
- 1 handful mint
- 1 handful parsley
- 1/2 cucumber, peeled and chopped
- 1 large celery stalk
- 1-inch piece of fresh ginger, peeled
- Juice of 1/2 a lemon
- Add a 1/2 apple, peach, or a handful of fresh pineapple if you need a li'l sweet

Blend all ingredients with ice until smooth and pour into a glass. Remember: ingredients are measured loosely to my taste. So if you love cucumber, include more cukes. And feel free to use whatever greens you have on hand like kale, chard, or lettuce leaves.

In addition to its yummy flavor, coconut water contains potassium and electrolytes, both of which are essential for staying hydrated during hard workouts. Coconut water is pure and natural—it's just the juice from inside the coconuts that grow all over Hawaii. Zico is my favorite brand. I surf for Zico, and they have a ton of fun flavors to try (though I gotta say the original is my fave!).

You may be wondering where soda falls into the realm of hydration. Hate to say it, but soda is a real no-no. In just one can of regular soda, there are ten teaspoons of sugar! Imagine yourself eating spoonfuls of sugar, one after the other. You wouldn't! So why drink all that sugar?

Some girls rely on diet soda to get a dose of sweetness sans the calories, but that includes artificial chemicals that have ample scientific research to make you cringe. Plus, it just makes you crave sugar later. Studies have linked soda to obesity, heart problems, and lower bone density (which means bones become more fragile in old age—not good). Why bother?

So what to sip instead of soda, especially when you need a little energy? Try hot or iced tea. I don't mean those bottles of sweetened tea that you can grab at the convenience store, but rather, pure tea you brew at home.

I like Tazo's Wild Sweet Orange and Passion teas, and Bengal Spice by Celestial Seasonings, which has cinnamon and ginger. Green tea has lots of antioxidants, which can protect your body from diseases. I also like mint tea (which is good for tummy aches), and some people find chamomile tea to be relaxing before bed. Whenever you have a craving for soda, try out teas instead. Soon enough you'll love a nice warm tea in the morning, on cold days, or in the evening, and iced tea in the summer rocks!

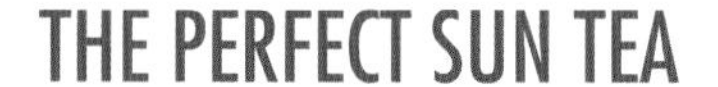

THE PERFECT SUN TEA

One of the easiest and best-tasting ways to enjoy tea of any flavor is to make sun tea. Fill a clear, glass pitcher with cold water, add a few tea bags, and place the pitcher in the sun. The sun naturally brews the tea. Let it sit in the sun for an hour, then grab a cup of ice and enjoy.

Great combo for summer sun tea:

- 1 teabag regular black tea
- 1 teabag green tea
- 1 teabag mint tea

BETHANY'S SOUL SECRET

A great way to relax at the end of the day? Brew a cup of tea and then sip it while writing in your journal. I'll add a dash of honey and a squeeze of lemon to an herbal tea, and it's just like a dessert.

"We're all created in God's image and can have faith that we're capable of doing anything we set our minds to."

—Bethany

CHAPTER 5

Surfer Secrets For Your Best Bod

(No Matter What)

I surf like it's my job because, well, it is. I'm blessed to be able to surf for a living, traveling all over the world to ride some epic waves and compete against some of the most amazing surfers out there.

So naturally, I've developed the body type—and healthy habits—that suit my lifestyle and my career. But even if you've never stepped foot on a board, or if you live hundreds of miles away from the ocean, you can still get your best bod.

When it comes to your body and your fitness, it's not just about having ripped abs or cut biceps—although those definitely don't hurt in surfing. It is more about getting your body to move more fluidly and having stability, power, and stamina to endure getting thrashed around the ocean by some pretty gnarly waves.

Every workout I do hits all of the major areas I need to utilize while surfing, whether it's my shoulders and my arm (for paddling out to the waves) or my legs (for keeping my feet firmly placed on the board and in control while I'm riding a twenty-foot swell).

My trainer, Dustin, has come up with an awesome approach to my fitness that has totally revamped the way I work out. Our major focus is posture, which helps me overcome a lot of balance and symmetry issues I have because of my missing arm.

Beyond that, by focusing on key principles like a strong upper body and core, better stability, agility, strength, and endurance, I'm fitter now than I've ever been—and I'd love to share our favorite moves with you.

CHECK YOUR HEAD

Whenever you go after a new goal—whether it's staying up on the surfboard or just being fit enough to run a mile—you've gotta start with the right mindset. Sure, you may love the idea of having six-pack abs, but are you 100 percent committed to stop at nothing 'til you get 'em?

Step number one is getting motivated to make it happen. Because there's no way you're going to be able to if you don't believe in yourself, right? When it comes to achieving my personal fitness goals, I need to have a ton of trust in my body. We're all created in God's image and can have faith that we're capable of doing anything we set our minds to.

I'm not going to sugarcoat it: Committing yourself to a workout program is no walk on the beach. But you can *totally* do it.

How do I know? Because you're tough. Think about it: As humans, we've survived for a ridiculously long time in some incredible circumstances, like famines and droughts. We're hardy, and capable of doing much more than we give ourselves credit for. We're definitely not fragile.

And we're hardwired for movement too. Everything in our body—from our immune system to our digestive system—requires movement in order to stay in tip-top shape. So that's why when you really get into an awesome flow with your fitness, you'll not only look amazing, but you'll *feel* amazing too.

GET UP, STAND UP (STRAIGHT)

Ever since I was just a tiny wahine, I've been active. I started surfing before I could read, and my natural athleticism made it easy for me to paddle out to the waves, hop up on the board, and hang on all the way to the shore.

Even though I was already starting to compete, it never felt like work. And how could it? I was having too much fun. After losing my arm, though, reality set in: Getting back to the top level of the surfing circuit meant regaining a ton of strength and balance so I could go out and ride those waves once again.

A major element of getting that surfer strength back was perfecting my posture. Because I was significantly stronger on my right side, my spine had started to curve in that direction. Yikes. After hearing that news, I headed straight to Dustin's office, and we got to work.

Just about every day, I do a bunch of exercises and stretches that focus on postural alignment—a fancy way of saying getting my body straight. Within three months of working with Dustin, my spinal alignment had shifted by 50 percent. Now *that's* progress. And for me it was a blessing!

Although my body is different than most girls, posture is super important for everyone. And a lot of us have big room for improvement. As Dustin says, spinal alignment and posture can have huge effects on your body's health. Did you know that poor posture can contribute to problems like headaches and stomach issues? Slouching actually presses your rib cage and organs against your lungs, resulting in less oxygen to your muscles.

So it doesn't matter if you are a soccer player, a surfer, or a swimmer—everything we do reacts to our posture. (Think about all the damage you do by lugging around that heavy backpack at school all day, not to mention poor posture sitting in class all day.)

That's why it's key to make your posture and spinal alignment a top priority. Thanks to Dustin, I've gained a deeper understanding of the human body's function and its relationship to correct posture. Need more incentive than just knowing you are standing up straight? I've got a ton more energy and almost never get sick anymore!

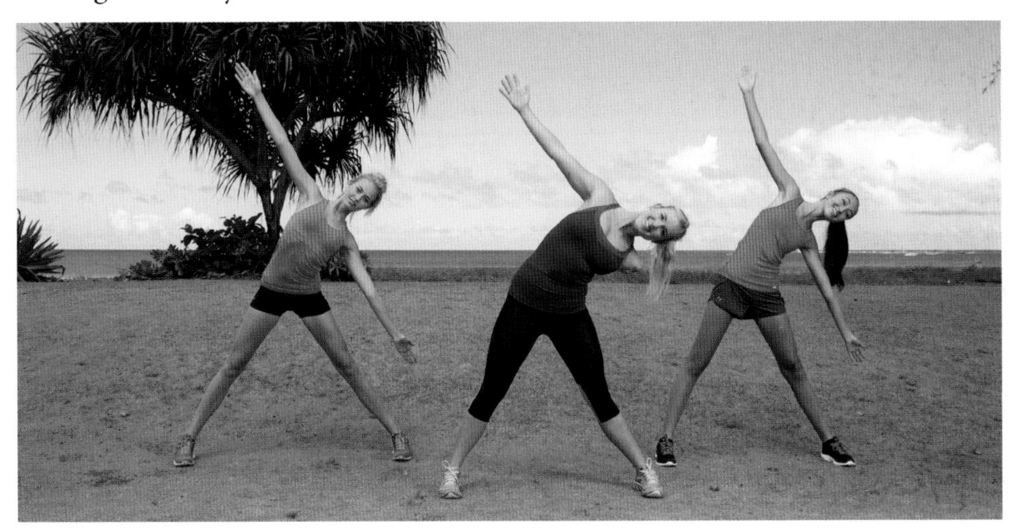

A SURFER'S STRENGTH

Aside from awesome posture, what else does it take to be an epic surfer? Swimming skills, for sure. And yeah, you've gotta have a healthy fear and respect for the ocean.

Despite what happened to me when I was thirteen, I still madly love the water, and I feel blessed that I get to go out and be a mermaid every single day. But beyond that, to compete among the world's best surfers, I have to focus my workouts on certain core components.

Because these components are so important to my training routine, I want to break down exactly what they are—and how they apply to you.

STABILITY This is all about having awesome form and overall balance. No matter if you're standing on a surfboard, swinging a golf club, or horseback riding, you've gotta make sure your body is stable and working in a fluid motion. Otherwise, you're pretty much asking for injury.

AGILITY On the ocean, I rely on my agility—the power to move quickly and easily—when I'm jumping up on my feet to surf or twisting my body from side to side. Every day, you need agility to react to potential hazards in your way, like saving yourself from completely wiping out in front of your whole school when you trip in the hallway. Totally key.

STRENGTH I'm not talking mega muscles here, but just being toned from head to toe so I can carve any wave that comes at me. Overall strength helps you kill it in any sport—and look fab.

ENDURANCE Paddling out to the waves and getting thrashed by swell after swell is no joke. I need a big engine to keep me going out there for hours. Whether you're running a 5K or tearing it up on the dance floor, having stamina keeps your motor running—and keeps you from quitting.

TAKE A POSTURE PICTURE

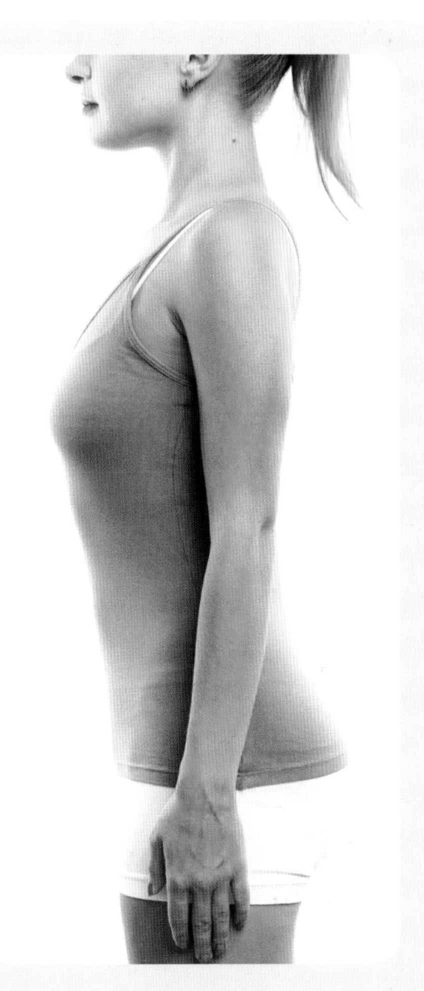

Not sure if your posture needs work? Here's an easy way to find out:

- Have one of your buds snap shots of you from the front, back, and side, standing as you normally do.
- Print out each pic on a separate sheet of paper.
- How do you tell if anything is off? For the front and back views, look to see if your arms are hanging differently (like one hand is lower than the other) or if your head or torso are slightly off to one side. For the side view, you should be able to draw a straight line from your ankle to your knees, hips, shoulders, and ear.
- If things aren't lining up, then it's time to focus on getting your alignment right. And as you do, make sure to take pictures every few months to see if you're improving that posture. Fun, right? Now you can see your progress!

NO WEIGHTS REQUIRED

Speaking of keeping your motor running, one of the things I love the most about training with Dustin is that all you really need is you and some motivation, not a ton of equipment.

I want to be fit, not ripped. Take a look at most surfer girls. Our body types are typically longer and lean versus big and bulky. Yeah, a lot of us rock some killer curves too, but you won't see any bulging biceps up on those boards. Healthy and toned is where it's at.

So, instead of grabbing the weights when working out, I use my own bodyweight as resistance. You'll see me using my TRX suspension training straps or doing a lot of moves like planks, tuck jumps, squats, pushups—all that require me to "lift" my body.

Study after study shows that bodyweight exercises are a quick and effective way to improve your balance, flexibility, and strength—which is basically everything I need to surf wrapped up in a pretty little package.

Don't get me wrong: every once in a while you may want to mix it up by swinging a kettlebell or doing a few reps with a light barbell. But I totally love the fact that you can get an amazing workout anywhere in the world and don't have to rely on any equipment. (Plus, who wants to spend tons of money on stuff if you don't have to?) All you've gotta have are the right moves, which we'll get to in just a bit.

STAY PURE

As you've probably figured out by now, I'm all about clean living. From the food I eat to the water I drink, I really try to keep my body pure as much as I can so I can stay healthy, active, and energetic.

Still, it's tough to totally steer clear of toxins—just walking down the street you can breathe in environmental pollutants like car exhaust, plus we're constantly coming into contact with random chemicals in our food, beauty products, and detergent.

Which is yet another reason I love to work out: exercise is a natural way to help detox your system. Who needs fancy cleanses when you can just go for a run? Because your blood circulates faster and more efficiently through the body when you exercise, it helps flush out toxins lurking in your system. I feel good when I work up a sweat!

Also, since you naturally take in more oxygen while you exercise, you can rid your lungs of carbon dioxide as you breathe in more oxygenated air.

In fact, with each heart-pounding workout you do, you're trashing a ton of toxins, which can bring you amazing benefits, like clearer skin and better digestion. Not to mention you can soak up even more benefits from sweating—another way to kick those icky toxins to the curb.

But it's not just exercise that can bring on those healthy vibes. Since deep breathing exercises and meditation also work to increase the amount of oxygen you take in, you get the same sort of benefits as working out. So even if you can't squeeze in a workout, starting your day with a prayer and some soulful deep breathing is *almost* just as good. Bonus if you can do both!

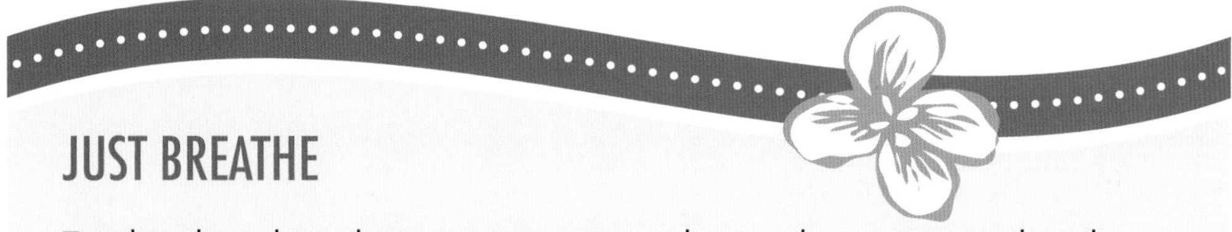

JUST BREATHE

Try this deep breathing exercise every day to clear your mind and increase the oxygen flow into your bod.

1. Toss a pillow on your floor and have a seat (you can also sit outside if it's not too cold).
2. Close your eyes and let your hands rest in your lap as you sit up straight.
3. Relax and concentrate on your breathing as you slowly inhale and exhale. As you breathe in, count to eight. As your breathe out, count to eight. Breathe in and out this way for a total of fifty times.
4. As you breathe, try to ignore any distracting thoughts. Thoughts will come; don't try to fight them. Instead, give them their moment, and then go back to focusing on your breathing. This will help clear your head of clutter.
5. When you hit fifty, take one last inhale and exhale, open your eyes, and stay seated for a couple more minutes as you stretch. Then stand up and get ready to face the day in the right frame of mind.

TIME TO SWEAT!

OK, so it's about that time to go out there and get your sweat on. Dustin and I have come up with four workouts based on the exercises I love. They'll each work you from head to toe while bringing you all sorts of extra benefits, like better balance, stability, posture, and endurance.

We recommend that you try these exercises at least three times a week (while mixing in other kinds of exercise, like hiking, tennis, basketball, or swimming) to keep you active every single day.

WORKOUT #1

SUPER STABILITY Looking to get long and lean? This workout is great for toning up since it burns fat and builds muscle too. Plus, it's awesome for getting better balance and strengthening your lower body. So whether you're trying to stay stable on a surfboard, kick harder on the soccer field, or nail that tree pose in yoga, this workout's totally for Y-O-U.

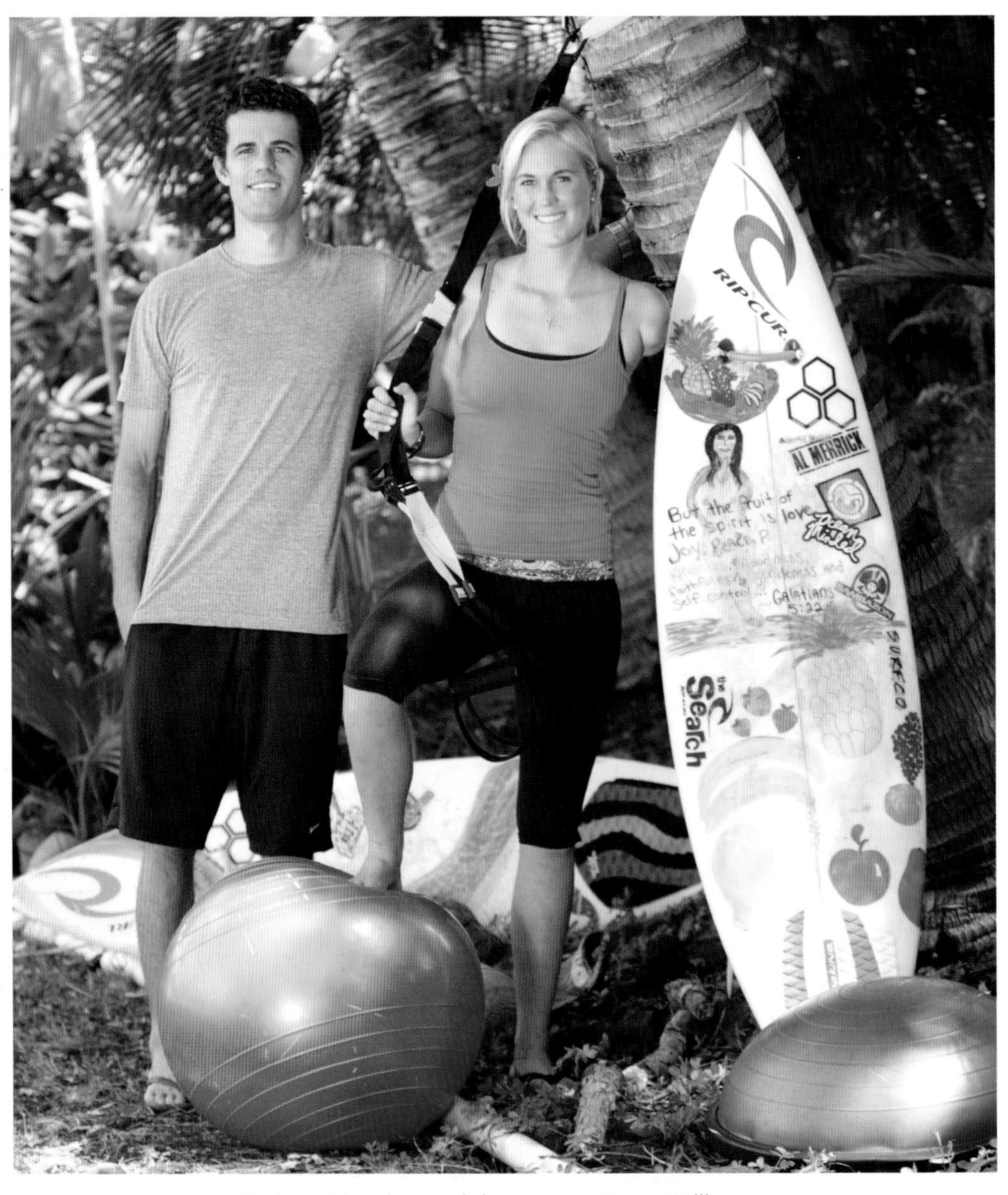

Bethany Hamilton with her trainer, Dustin Dillberg.

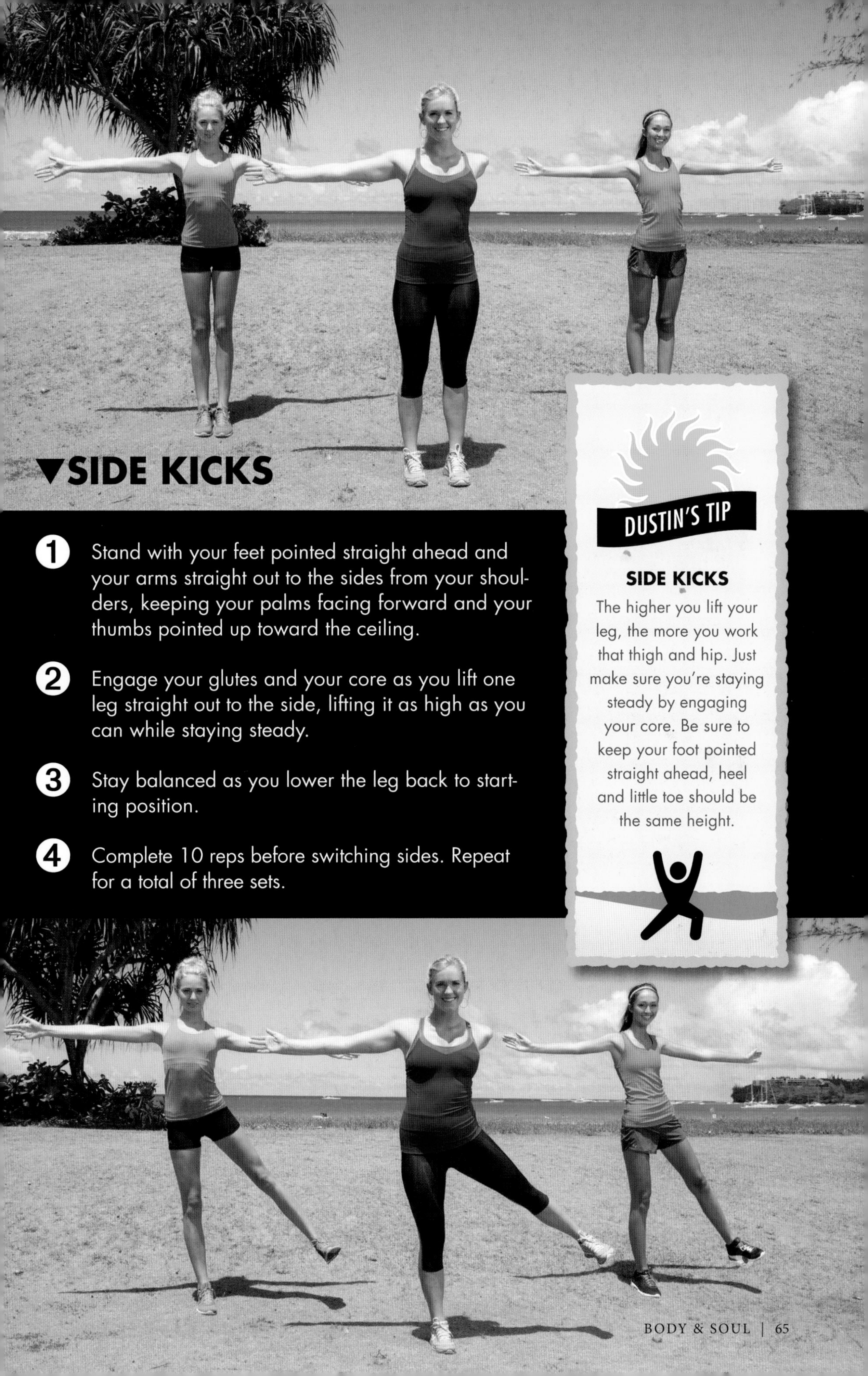

▼SIDE KICKS

1. Stand with your feet pointed straight ahead and your arms straight out to the sides from your shoulders, keeping your palms facing forward and your thumbs pointed up toward the ceiling.

2. Engage your glutes and your core as you lift one leg straight out to the side, lifting it as high as you can while staying steady.

3. Stay balanced as you lower the leg back to starting position.

4. Complete 10 reps before switching sides. Repeat for a total of three sets.

DUSTIN'S TIP

SIDE KICKS

The higher you lift your leg, the more you work that thigh and hip. Just make sure you're staying steady by engaging your core. Be sure to keep your foot pointed straight ahead, heel and little toe should be the same height.

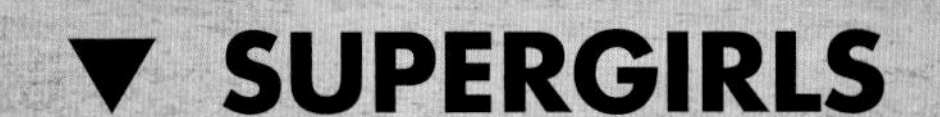

▼ SUPERGIRLS

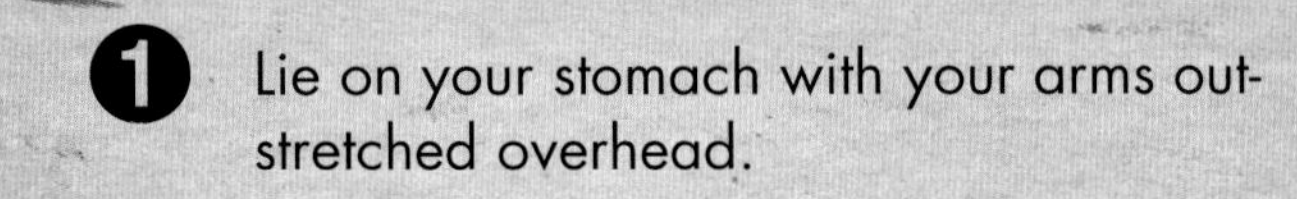

1. Lie on your stomach with your arms outstretched overhead.

2. Simultaneously lift your arms/hands and legs/feet about six inches off the floor. It should feel as if you are lifting and reaching forward with the arms, backward with the legs.

3. Hold for five to 10 seconds before returning back to your starting position; repeat for a total of six Supergirls.

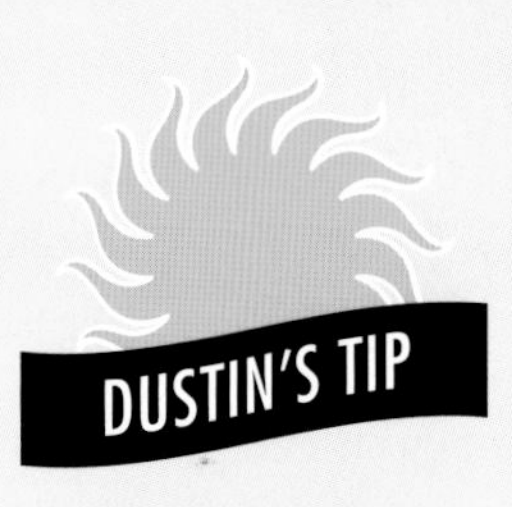

DUSTIN'S TIP

SUPERGIRLS:

Avoid overextending your back by pinching your heels together, which will keep your glutes engaged.

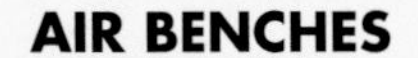

AIR BENCHES

This move is super challenging, so if you find this too hard at first, slowly build your way up to two minutes. Ready to step it up? Lift your toes off the ground so you're on your heels.

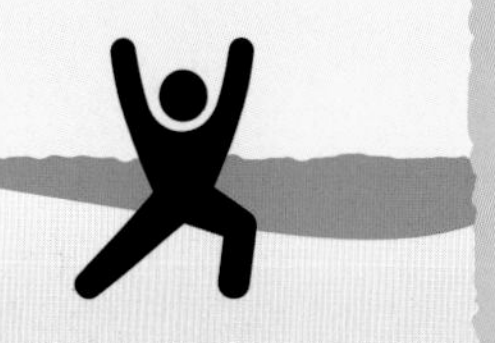

AIR BENCHES ►

1. Stand with your back against a firm surface with your feet and knees hip width apart and feet pointed straight.

2. Walk your feet away from the wall while sliding your body down at the same time, like you're sitting in an invisible chair. If you can, bend your knees to a 90-degree angle, but make sure your knees don't go past your toes. Keep your lower back completely flat against the wall, with all of your weight in your heels.

3. Hang your arms down by your sides or rest them on your lap while you hold the seated position for two minutes.

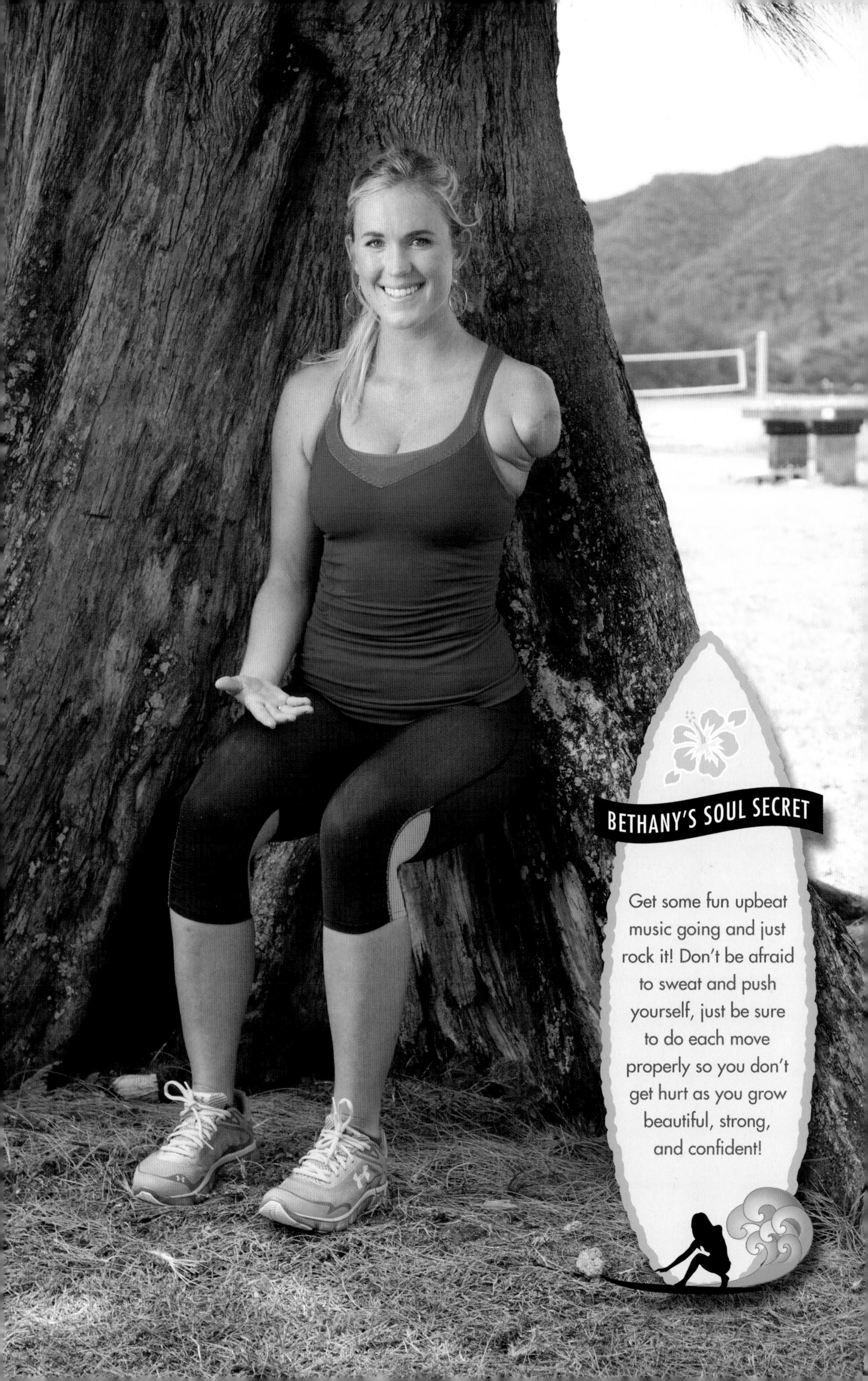
BETHANY'S SOUL SECRET
Get some fun upbeat music going and just rock it! Don't be afraid to sweat and push yourself, just be sure to do each move properly so you don't get hurt as you grow beautiful, strong, and confident!

▼ THIGH THINNERS

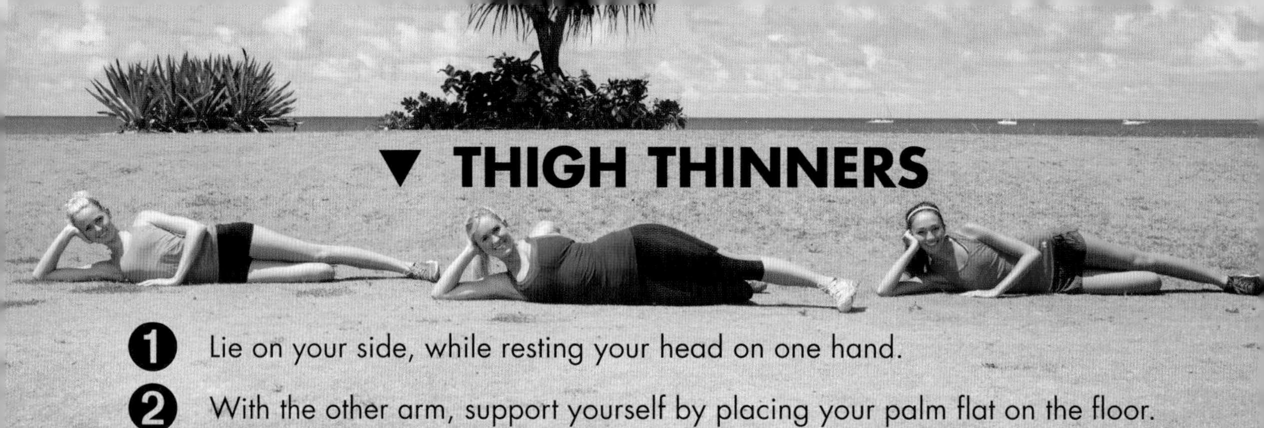

1. Lie on your side, while resting your head on one hand.
2. With the other arm, support yourself by placing your palm flat on the floor.

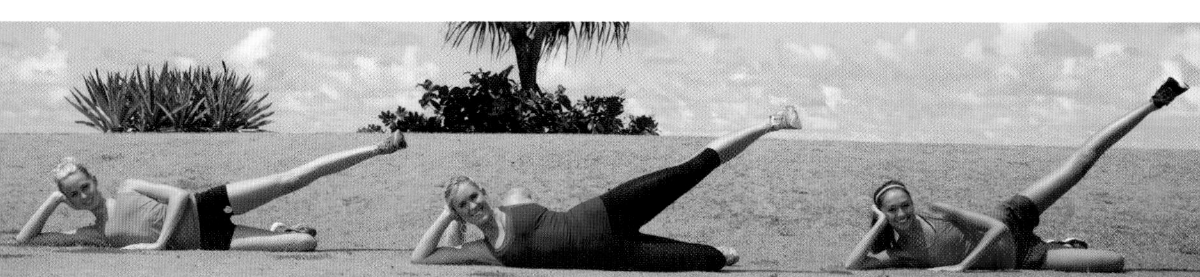

3. Bend your bottom leg so it's resting on the ground behind you, at about a 45-degree angle.
4. Hold the top leg straight, with your thigh tight and your foot flexed.

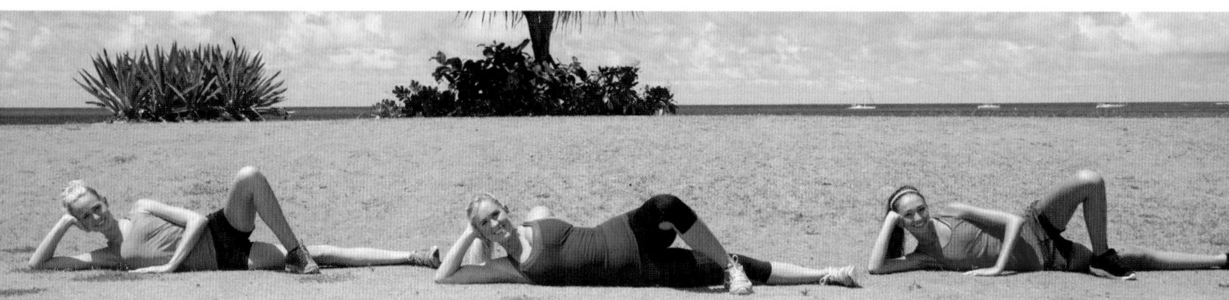

5. Slowly raise and lower the top leg for a total of 20 reps.
6. Switch legs by bending the top leg and placing your foot flat on the floor in front of you.

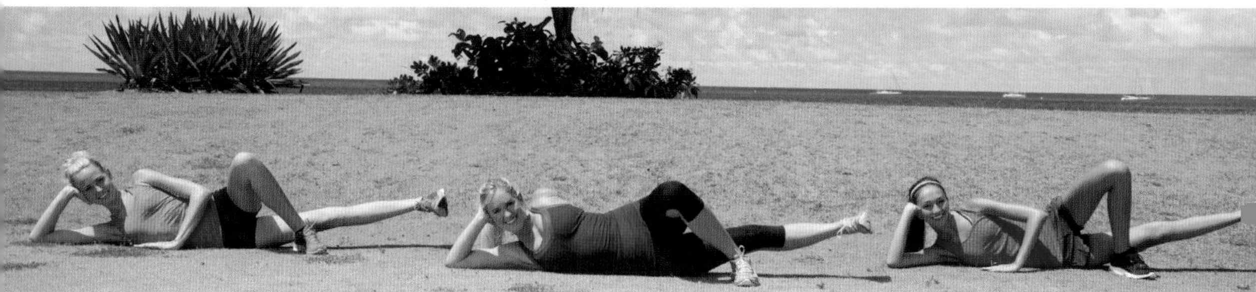

7. Straighten your bottom leg, and raise and lower it three to four inches off the floor, keeping your thigh tight and your toes flexed. Repeat for 20 reps.
8. Roll to the other side and repeat the entire sequence.
9. Do a total of three sets.

THIGH THINNERS

Be sure to target the muscles around the hips rather than muscles in your back and stomach.

JUMP FOR JOY

Make sure to use your whole foot to jump, not just your toes. This will give you more explosive power. Push yourself!

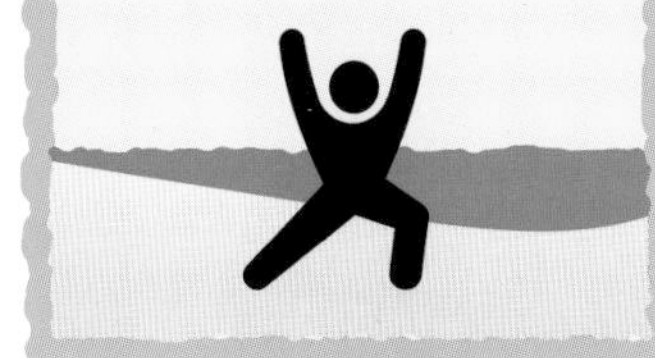

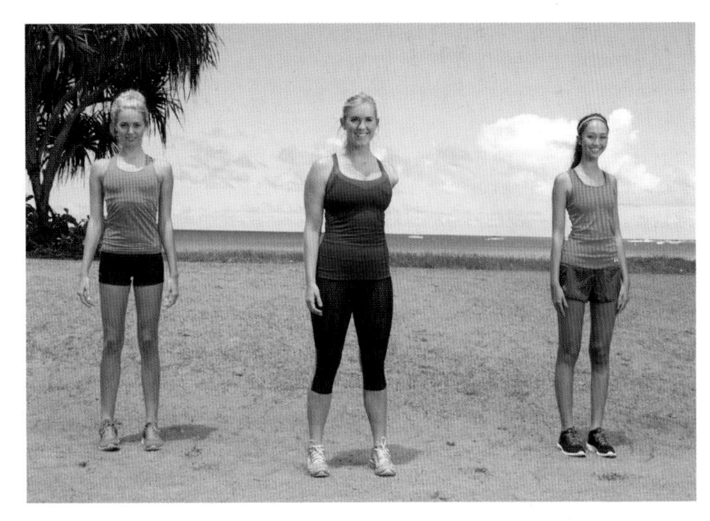

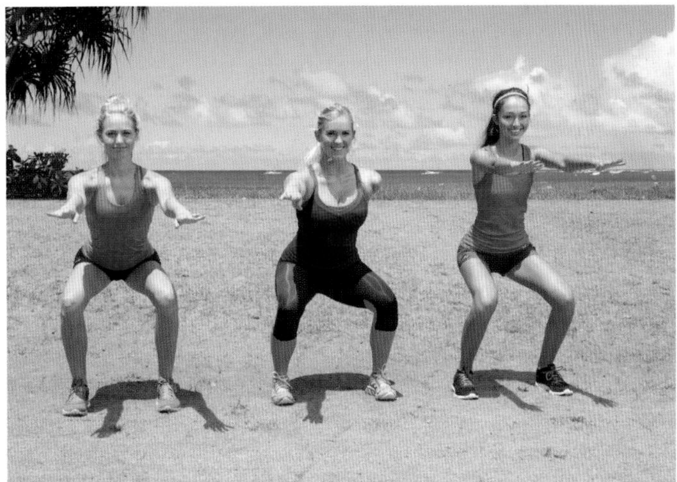

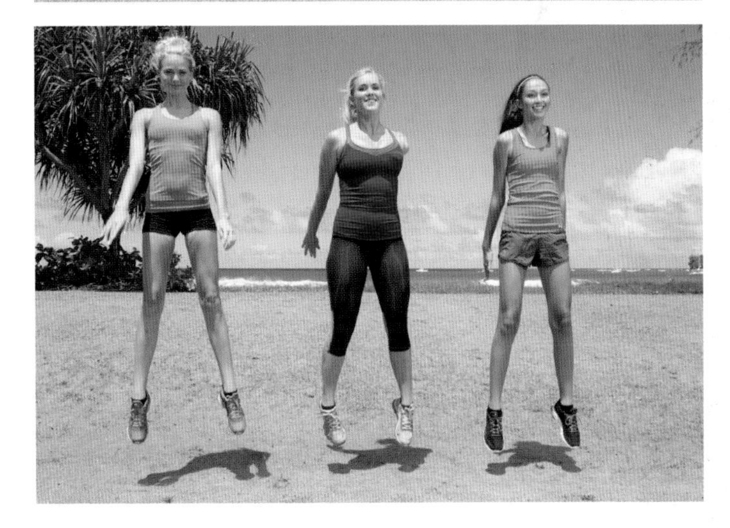

JUMP FOR JOY

1. Stand with your feet shoulder-width apart and rest your hands on your hips (I hold my hand straight out for balance instead of holding my hips).
2. Start by doing a regular squat, then jump up while engaging your core.
3. When you land, lower your body back into the squat position. That's one rep.
4. Do two sets of 10 reps.

WORKOUT #2

POSTURE UP! Having great posture not only keeps you injury-free, but it's also key for sports like swimming—and looking gorgeous in halter tops and sundresses. These moves will help you get your spinal alignment in check while offering up some bonus core and lower body boosts.

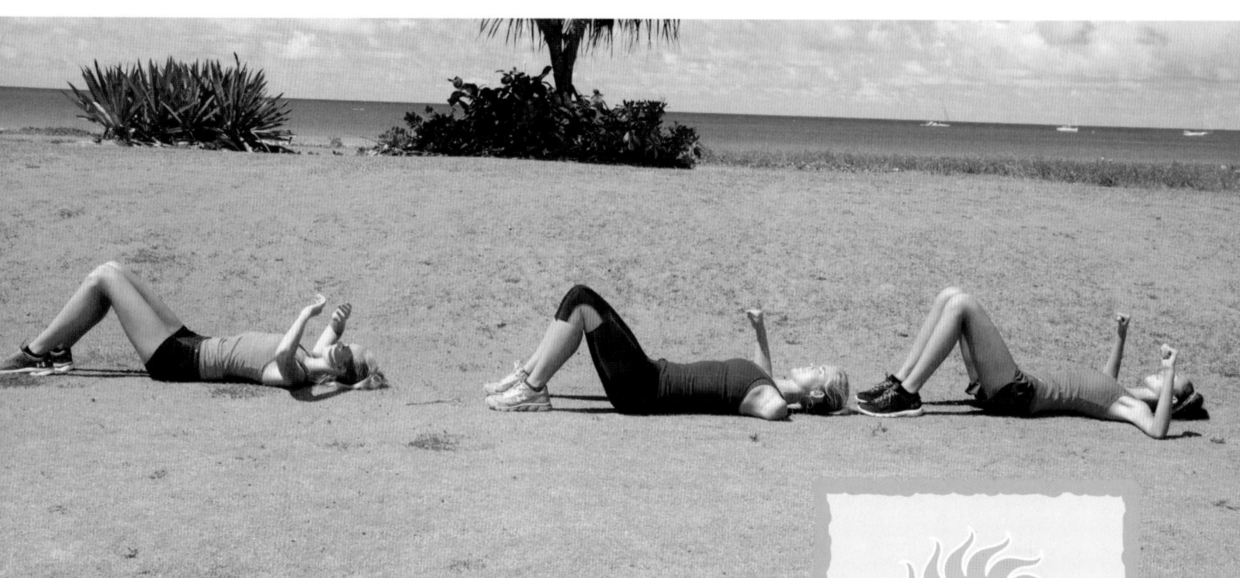

▲ PINCHERS

1. Lie on your back. To make this more difficult, put your legs up on a chair or ottoman.
2. With your arms out to the side, bend your elbows so your fists are up toward the sky.
3. Squeeze your shoulder blades down and together, holding the squeeze for one second, and then release.
4. Repeat for three sets of 10 squeezes.

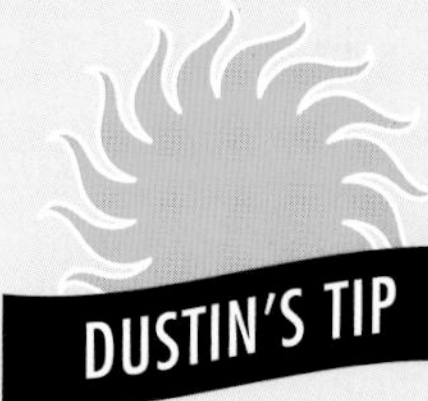

DUSTIN'S TIP

PINCHERS

While doing this move, think about pulling the bottom of your shoulder blades toward each other, then pressing your shoulder into the ground. Your elbows will stay relaxed on the ground.

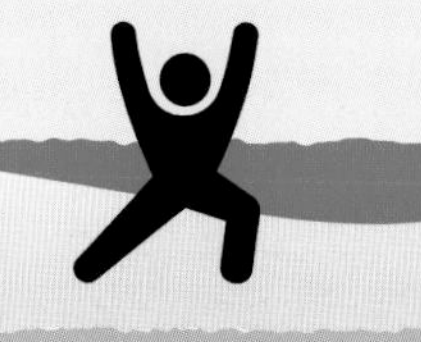

STANDING WINDMILLS

Keep your hips locked in place by imagining that they're super-glued to a wall. Only your upper body should move.

Do all you can to keep your neck and traps (muscles connecting shoulder to neck) relaxed through this whole exercise. If you notice them tensing up, pause and relax them before continuing.

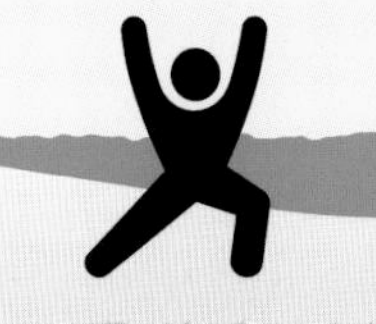

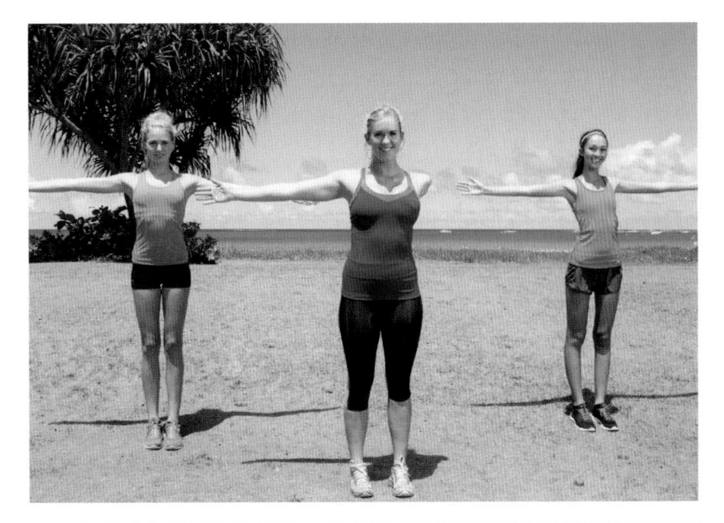

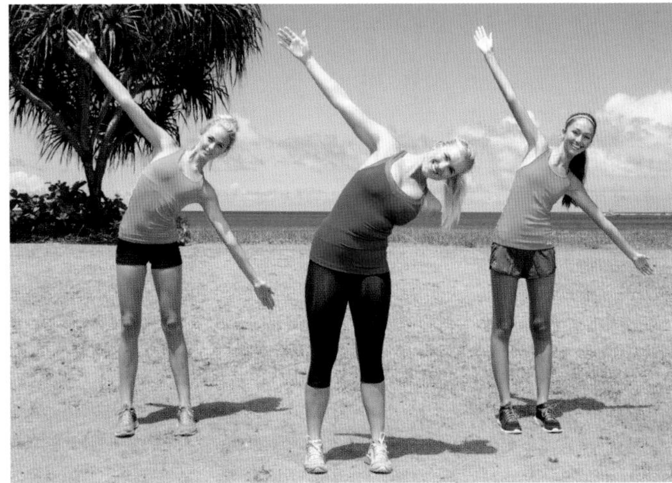

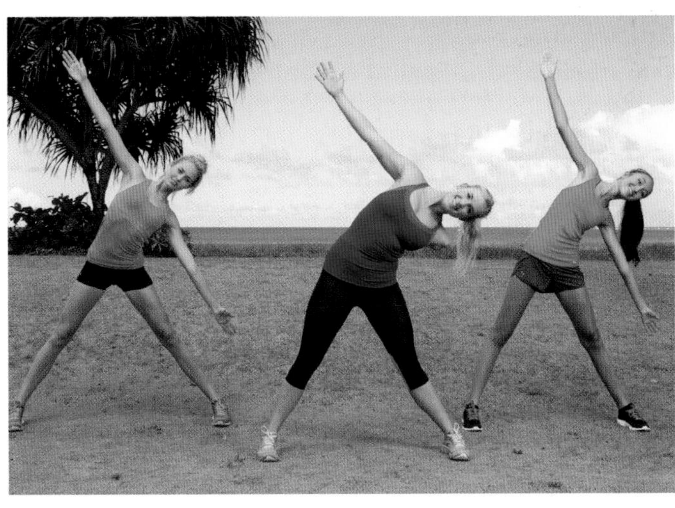

STANDING WINDMILLS ►

1. Start with your feet hip-width apart, arms out to the side, keeping them still and locked.
2. Slowly bend your torso to one side, then the other for five reps each direction.
3. Repeat steps one and two with your feet repositioned at 1½ feet apart, then 2½ feet apart, and then go back to hip-width apart for a total of 20 reps.

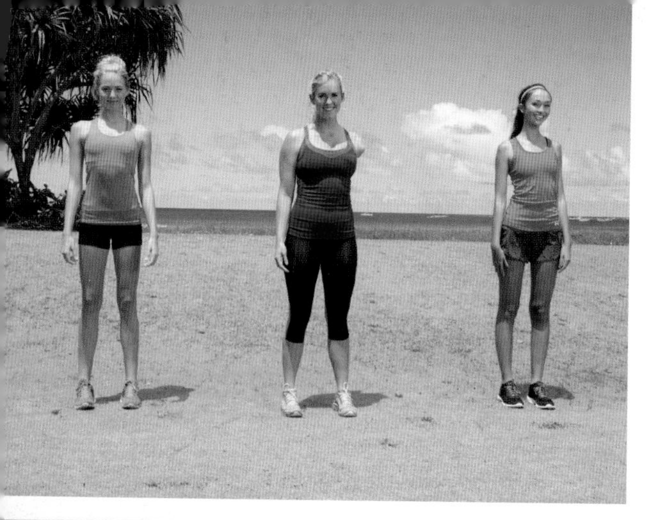

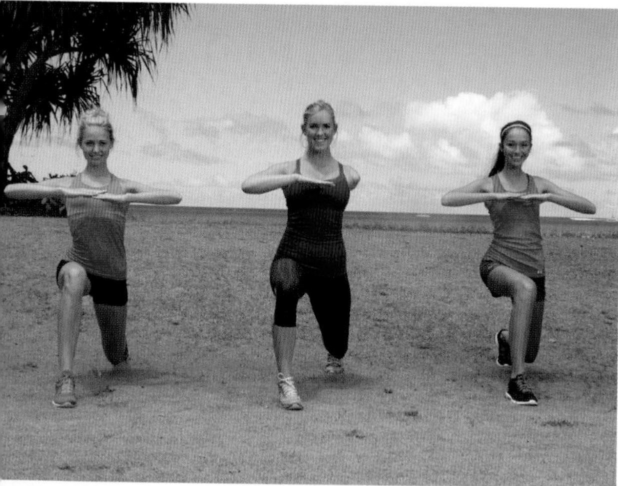

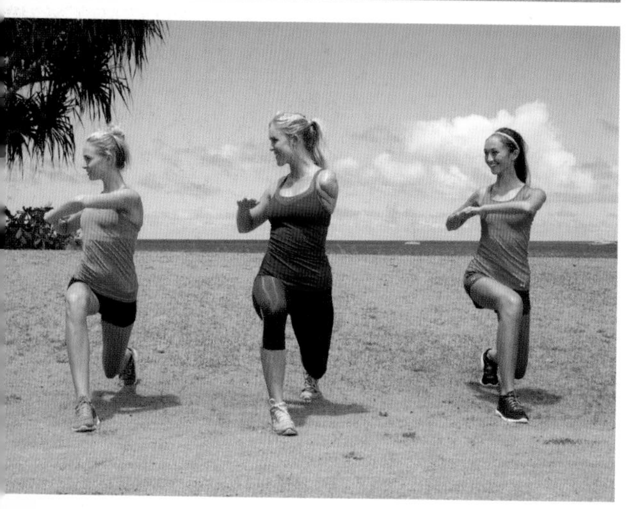

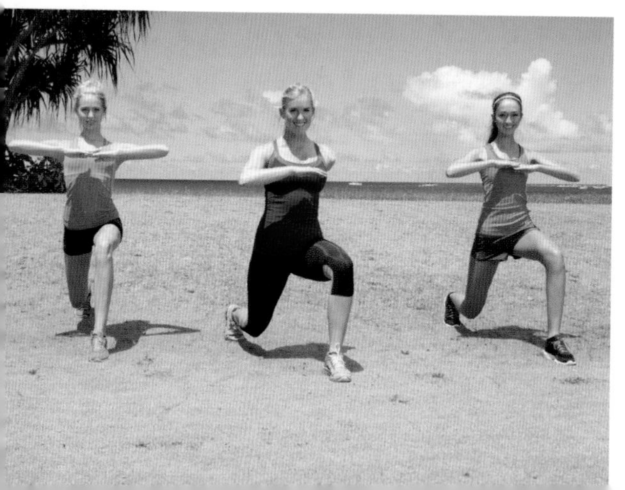

TWISTERS

1. Start in a standing position.
2. Step backwards into a lunge with your left foot, squeezing your left glute.
3. Twist your upper body over the front leg by taking your left elbow to the outside of the right knee.
4. Reverse the twist back to neutral and return to a standing position by pulling through with your left hip, and immediately stepping into a lunge with the other leg.
5. Continue for 10 reps before switching sides; repeat for two sets of 10 reps on each leg.

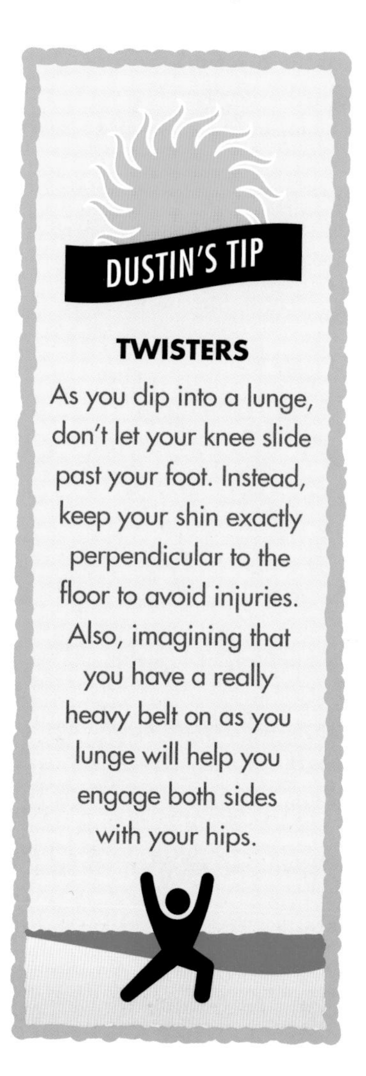

DUSTIN'S TIP

TWISTERS

As you dip into a lunge, don't let your knee slide past your foot. Instead, keep your shin exactly perpendicular to the floor to avoid injuries. Also, imagining that you have a really heavy belt on as you lunge will help you engage both sides with your hips.

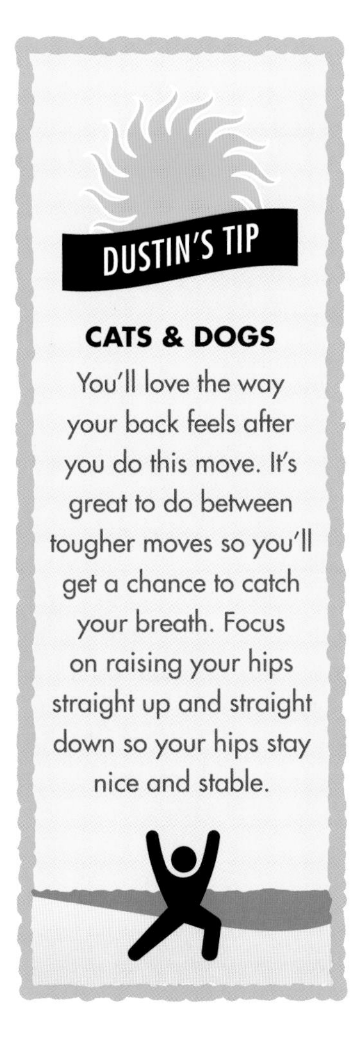

DUSTIN'S TIP

CATS & DOGS

You'll love the way your back feels after you do this move. It's great to do between tougher moves so you'll get a chance to catch your breath. Focus on raising your hips straight up and straight down so your hips stay nice and stable.

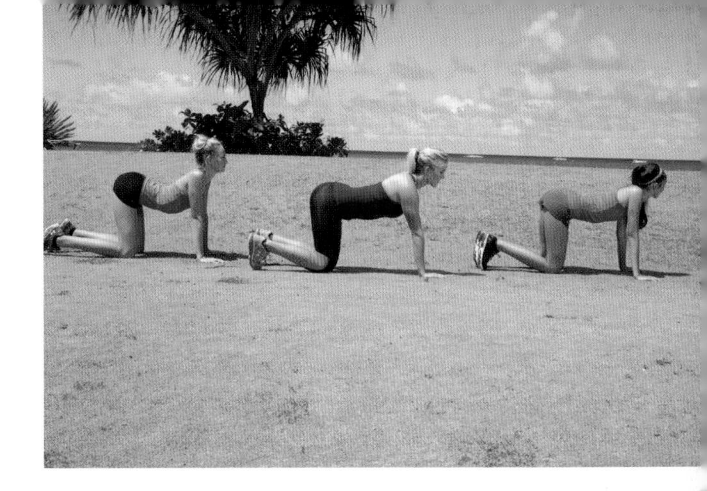

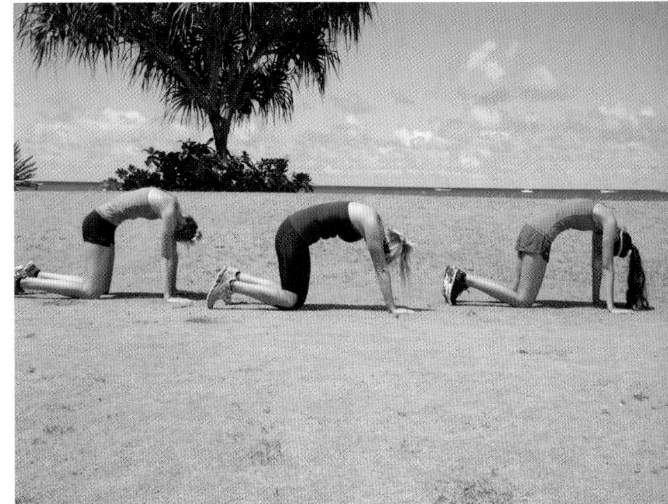

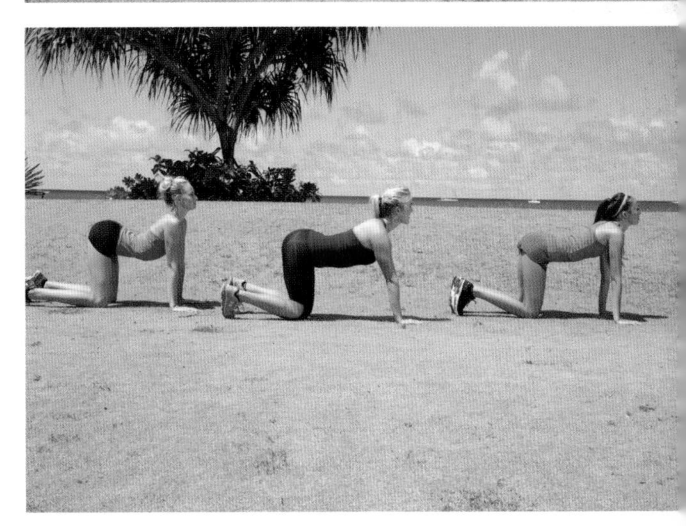

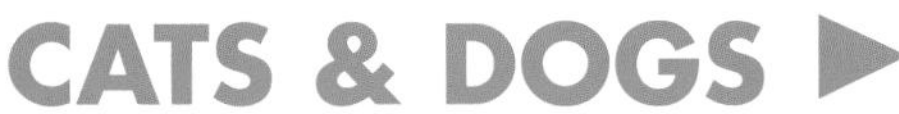

CATS & DOGS ►

1. Start on your hands and knees. Make sure your hips are directly above your knees, and your shoulders are directly above your hands. Your fingers should be pointed forward.
2. For the Cat position: Pull your hips under, pull your head under, and push your upper back to the ceiling to round your back up high.
3. For the Dog position: Roll your hips forward to put an arch in your back, collapse your shoulder blades together, and look up.
4. Slowly move back and forth between the Cat and Dog positions.
5. Repeat for a total of 10 Cats and 10 Dogs.

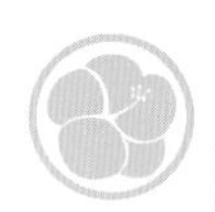

WORKOUT #3

AWESOME AGILITY

These moves are perfect for when I'm traveling and can't get in the ocean, but want to keep muscles toned and ready for when I get back on my board. Being low to the ground like this mimics being on a surfboard, plus it challenges the range of motion in your hips, which is key for riding the waves.

▼ SURFER BURPEES

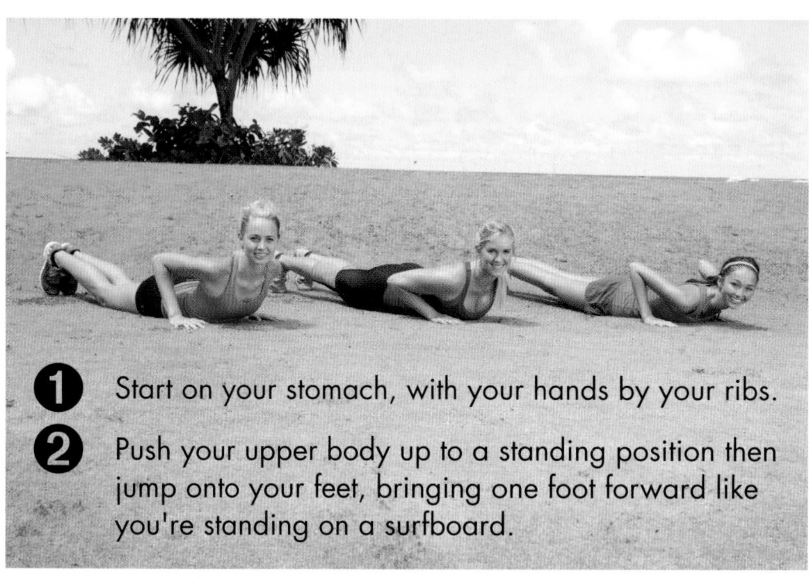

1. Start on your stomach, with your hands by your ribs.
2. Push your upper body up to a standing position then jump onto your feet, bringing one foot forward like you're standing on a surfboard.

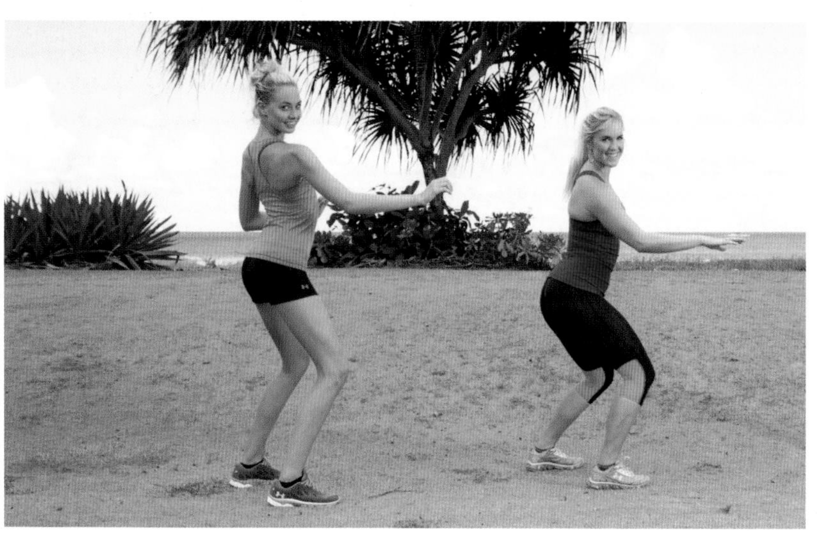

3. Jump up with your hands in the air, then immediately return to the starting position.
4. Repeat, alternating sides for as many times as you can in 30 seconds.

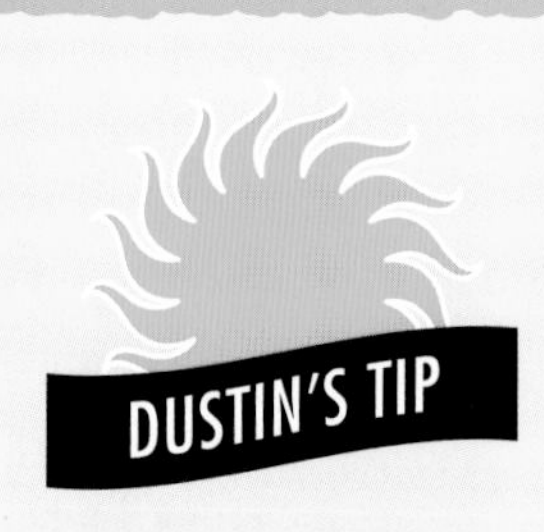

SURFER BURPEES

If you want to push yourself harder, add a jump squat. Once you're up, do a squat and jump. When you land, get back down. Switch sides as you go.

TUMMY CRUSHERS

Feel the burn. If your hips aren't screaming at you as you do this, you're not doing it right. If you're not quite ready to go up on your arm, try this from your elbow instead. And instead of having your leg completely straight out, go on your knees.

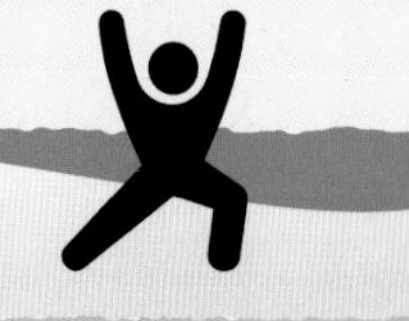

▼ TUMMY CRUSHERS

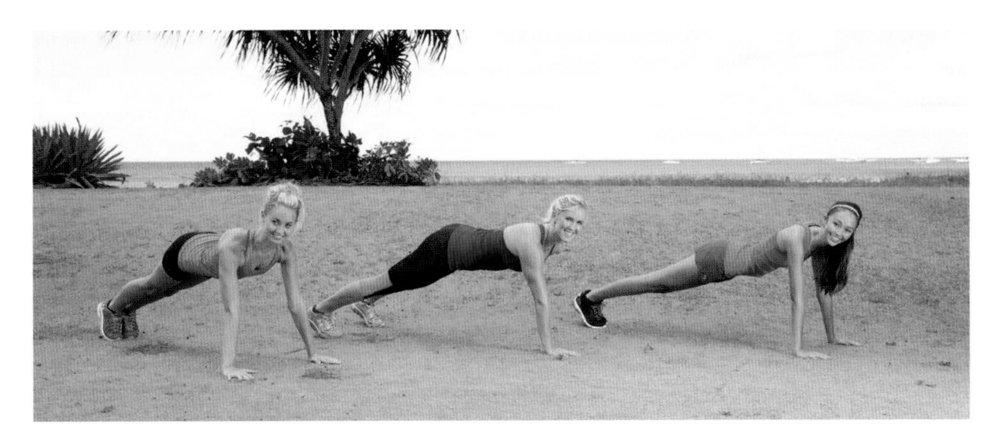

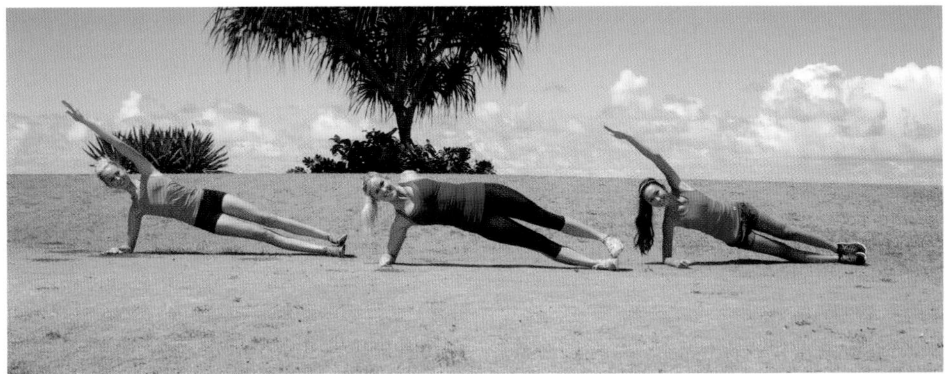

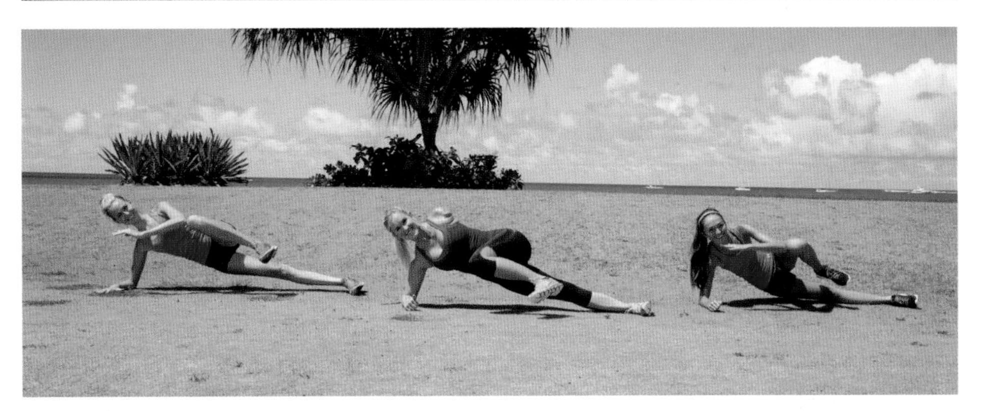

1. Start in a plank position with your arms straight and your shoulders over your wrists.
2. Roll over to your right side, balancing with your right hand right (under your shoulder) and the outside edge of your right foot.
3. Place your left (top) arm on your head with your elbow pointing towards the sky.
4. Bending your left (top) knee, slowly bring it toward your elbow. That's one rep.
5. Continue for 15 reps, then switch sides. Repeat for two reps on each side.

▼ DUCK WALKS

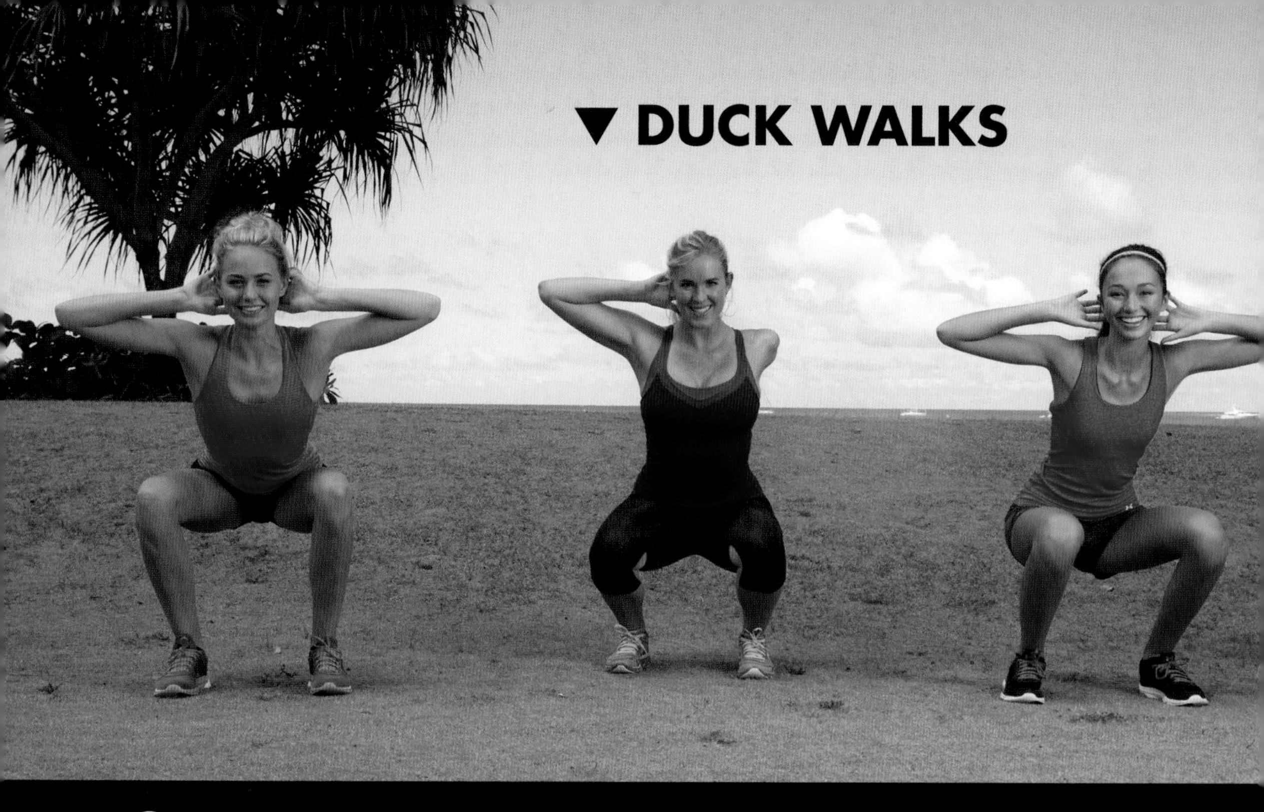

1. Stand with your feet hip-width apart.
2. Keeping your back straight and abs engaged, squat down until your thighs are parallel to the ground.
3. Keep your arms out for balance. Staying in the squat position, take one "duck walk" step by picking up your right calf and placing your foot flat on the ground in front of you.
4. Walk 10 alternating steps in a row.

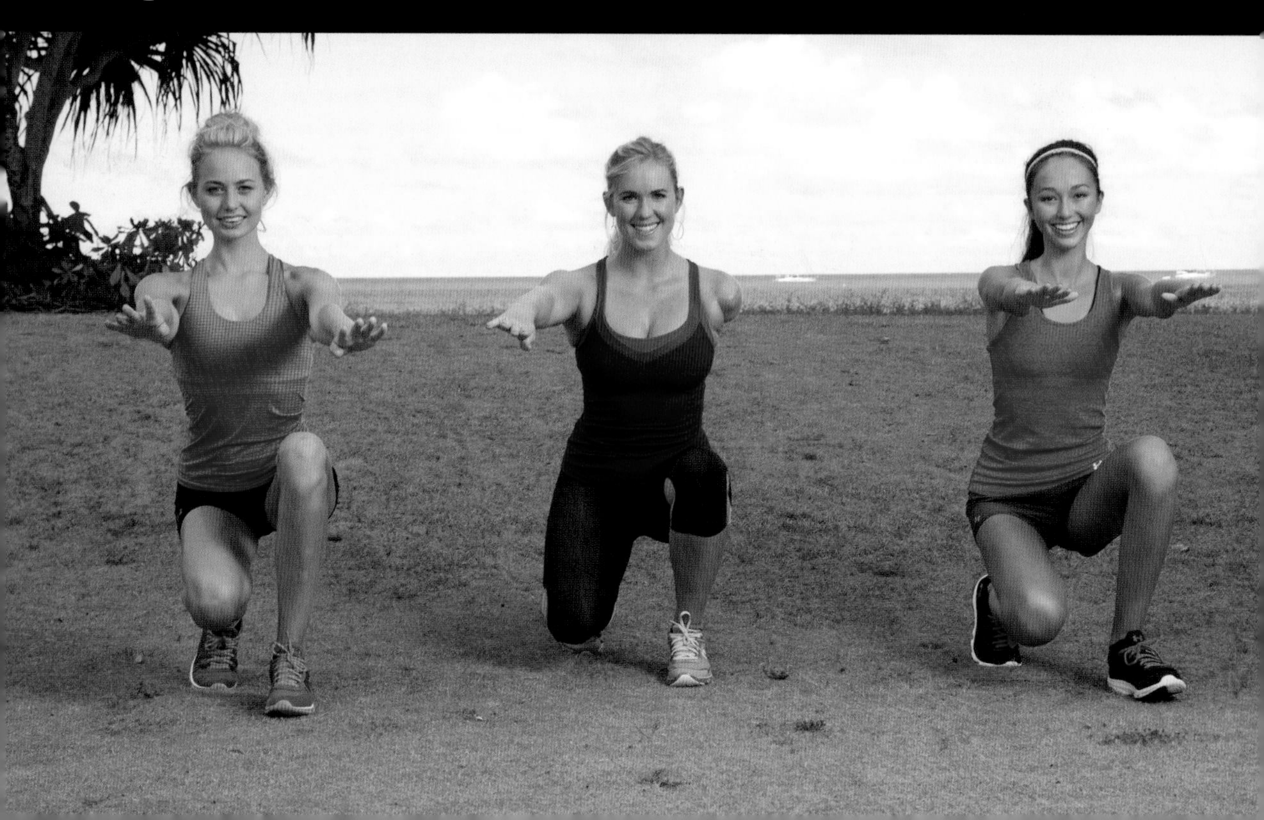

DUCK WALKS

Don't let your knees buckle while you walk to make sure you're not setting yourself up for injury.

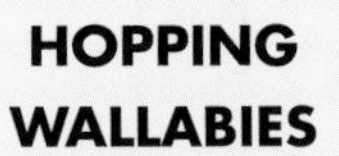

HOPPING WALLABIES

Hop as high as you can while staying in control, and landing with your feet in the same position as you started. Keep that smile on even when you start to feel the gain not pain!

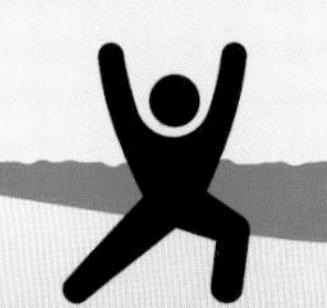

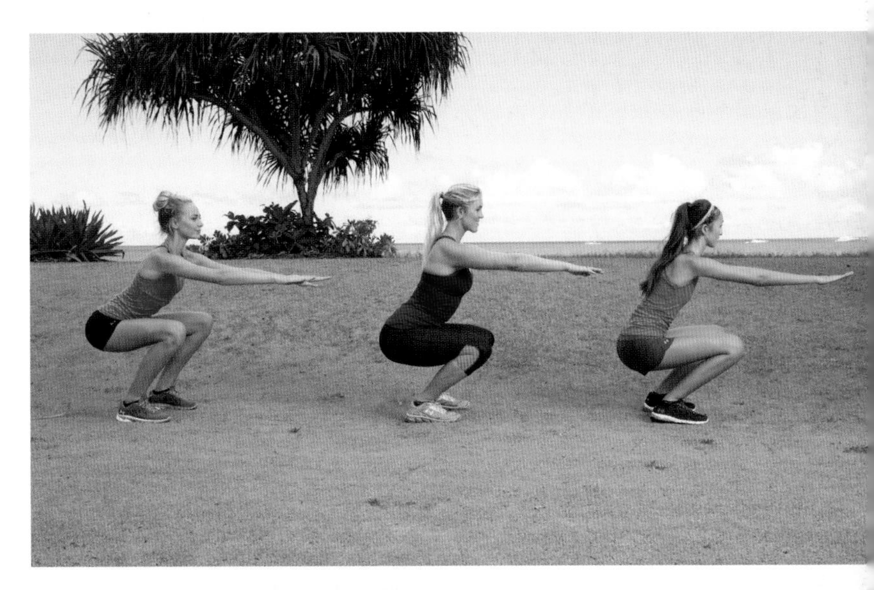

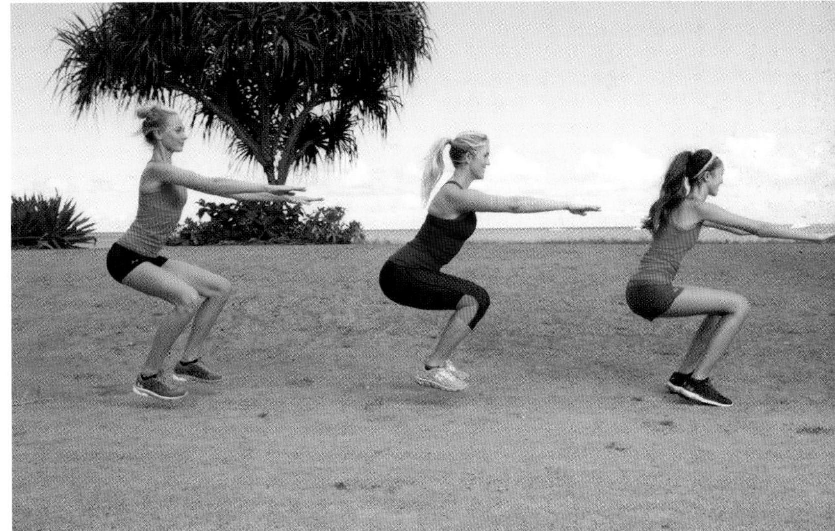

▲ HOPPING WALLABIES

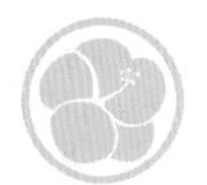

1. Get in a low squat position and reach your arms out in front of you for balance.
2. Rising up on your toes, do little jumps forward, making sure to keep your knees aligned with your hips.
3. Hold your stomach in and pull your shoulders back as you jump.
4. Repeat for 10 jumps.

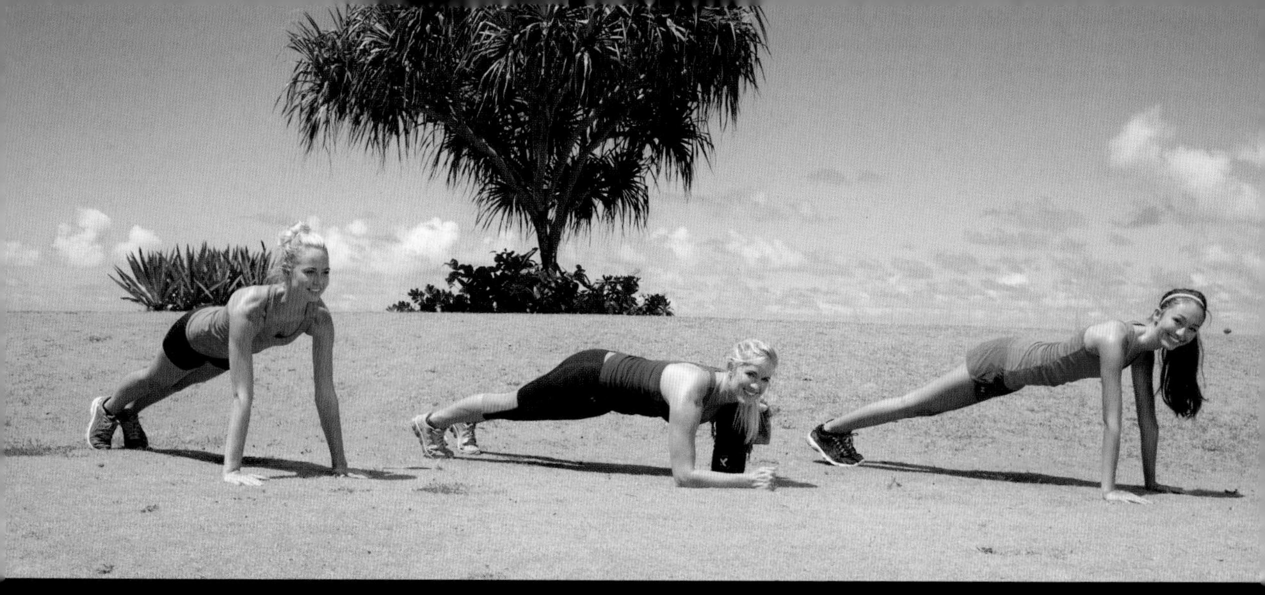

GRASSHOPPERS

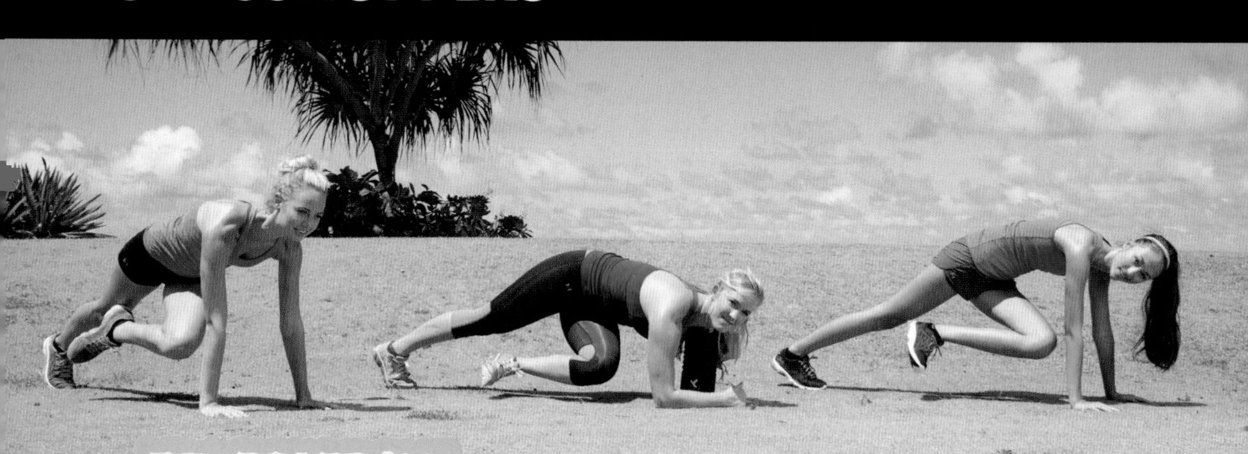

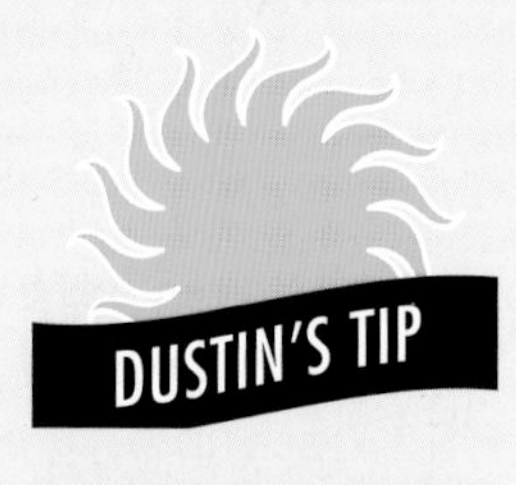

DUSTIN'S TIP

GRASSHOPPERS

Keep hips stable and glutes engaged as you move. To make it easier, just drive your knees straight up instead of toward your elbows.

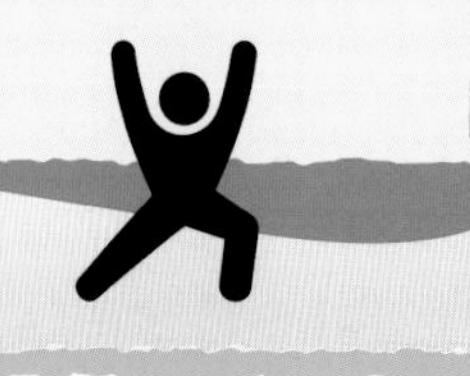

1. Start in a push-up position.
2. Keep your back flat and your hips facing the floor as you bend your right knee and bring it toward your right elbow.
3. Return your right leg to the starting spot and repeat with your left leg.
4. Do three sets of 20 reps, alternating sides.

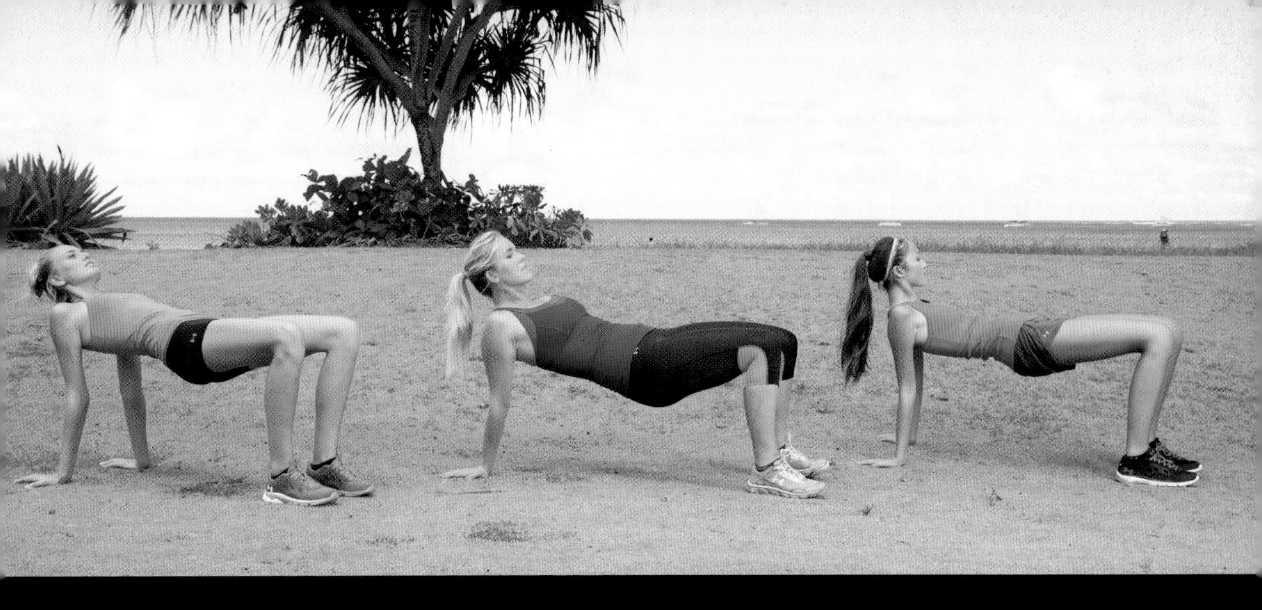

DANCING CRABS

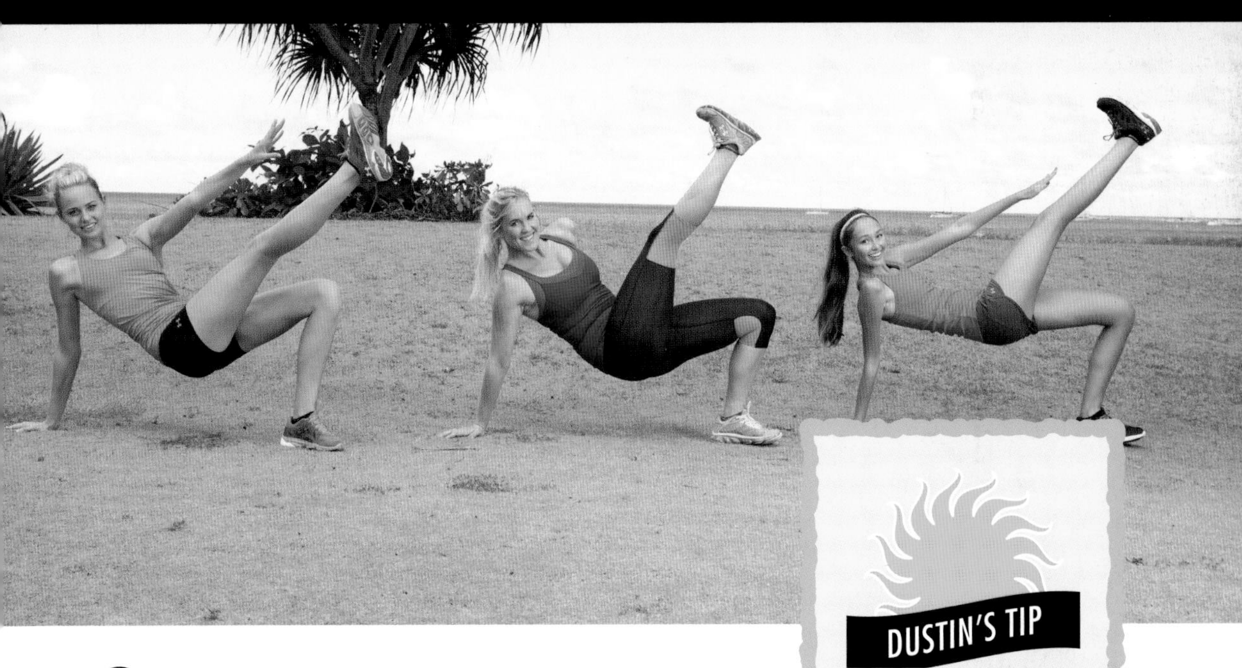

1. Get into a crab position, balancing on your hands and feet with your front facing the ceiling and your hips pointed up.

2. While lifting your right foot, lift your left hand and reach for your foot.

3. Return to starting position, then switch sides, reaching for your left foot with your right hand. That's one rep.

4. Complete two sets of 15 reps.

DUSTIN'S TIP

DANCING CRABS

Stay stable by keeping the supporting shoulder pulled down and back. Also, squeeze your glutes and lift your hips as high off the ground as you can to get the most out of this move.

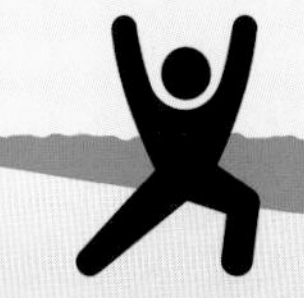

WORKOUT #4

SPEED PLAY

These moves get your heart rate going and your competitive fires burning as you race the clock.

HIGH KNEES

1. Start by raising your arms straight out in front of you, holding your shoulder blades back.
2. Lift your knees upward, alternating your feet at a quick pace.
3. Complete as many knee raises as you can in 30 seconds. Rest for 30 seconds and repeat for a total of two sets.

DUSTIN'S TIP

HIGH KNEES

Work on lifting from the front of your hips and making sure you're driving your knees straight up to the same side shoulder rather than across.

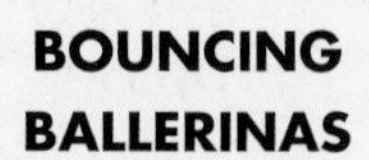

BOUNCING BALLERINAS

As you "explode up" drive with your hips and use your glutes to create more power than just your quads. This should make your heels gently come together.

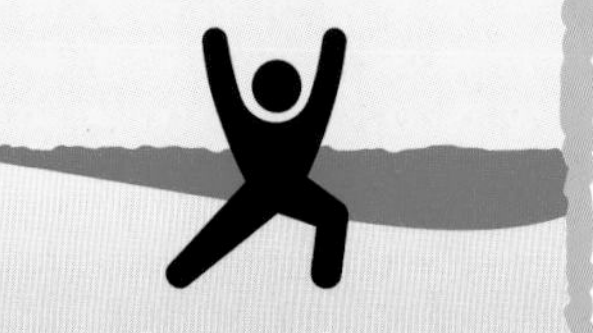

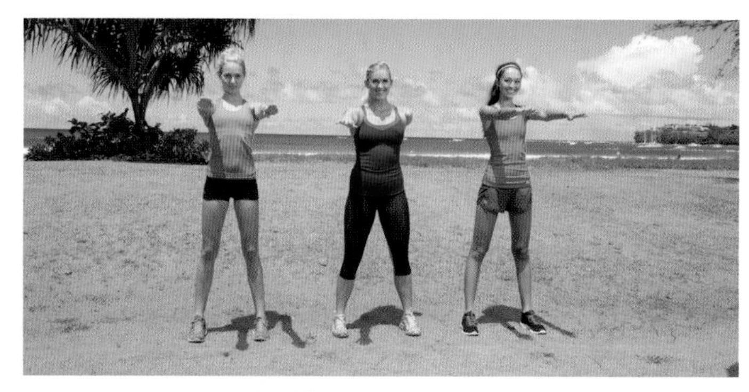

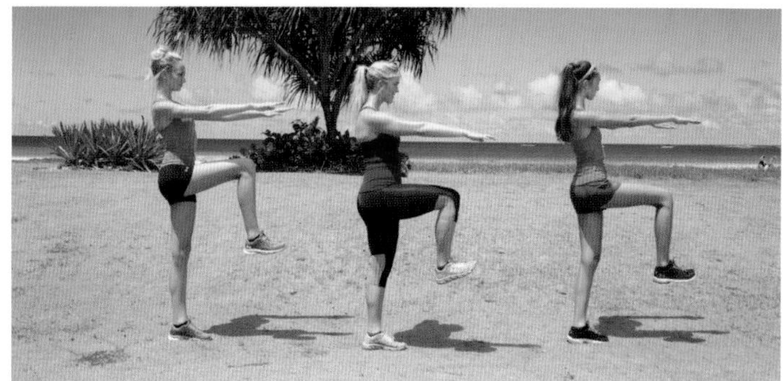

BOUNCING BALLERINAS

1. Start standing with your feet pointed straight ahead hip-width apart.
2. Control your movement as you lower yourself down into a nice low squat. Once at the bottom of the squat, explode up and jump as high as you can.
3. As you're in the air, click your heels together, then land back in your starting position.
4. Complete as many jumps as you can in 30 seconds. Rest for 30 seconds then repeat for a total of two sets.

NINJA TUCK JUMPS

1. Start on your knees in a kneeling "ninja" position.
2. Squeeze your glutes and quads as you explode up and jump to your feet.
3. Once on your feet, jump as high as you can and pull your knees up toward your chest.
4. Complete as many jumps as you can in 30 seconds, rest, then repeat for a total of two sets.

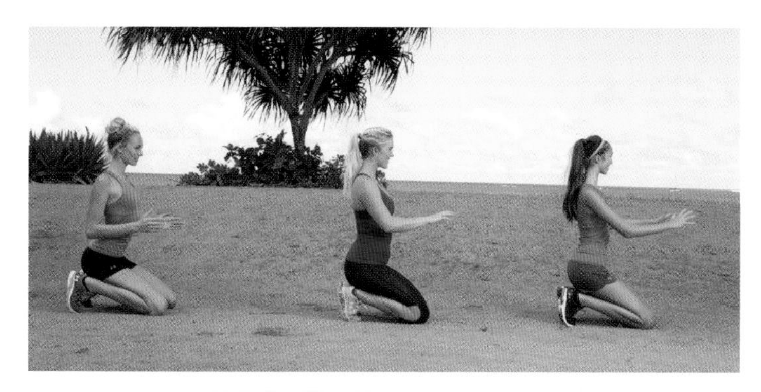

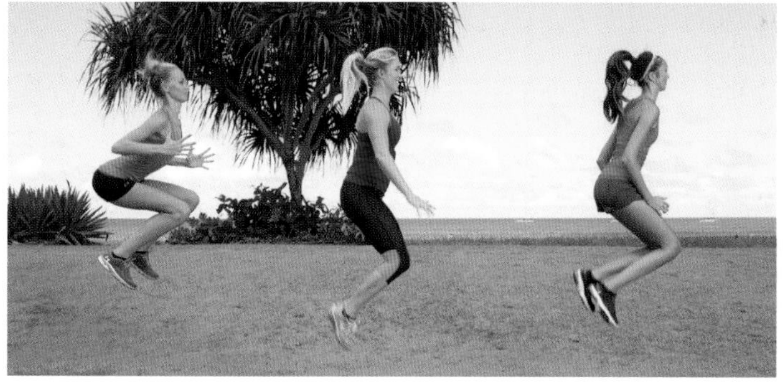

DUSTIN'S TIP

HILL SPRINTS

When doing sprints, always go for time, not distance. If you feel like you need more of a challenge, increase the time you're running hard by 10 seconds. Don't have a hill nearby? Run the stairs instead.

NINJA TUCK JUMPS

Really focus on your form here, making sure you're jumping and landing off of your right and left sides equally.

HILL SPRINTS

1. Find a hill close to your house.
2. Starting at the bottom of the hill, run as fast as you can until you reach the top (or for 30 seconds, whichever comes first).
3. When the time is up (or you reach the top), jog down to the bottom.
4. Once you reach your starting point, repeat for eight to 10 sprints.

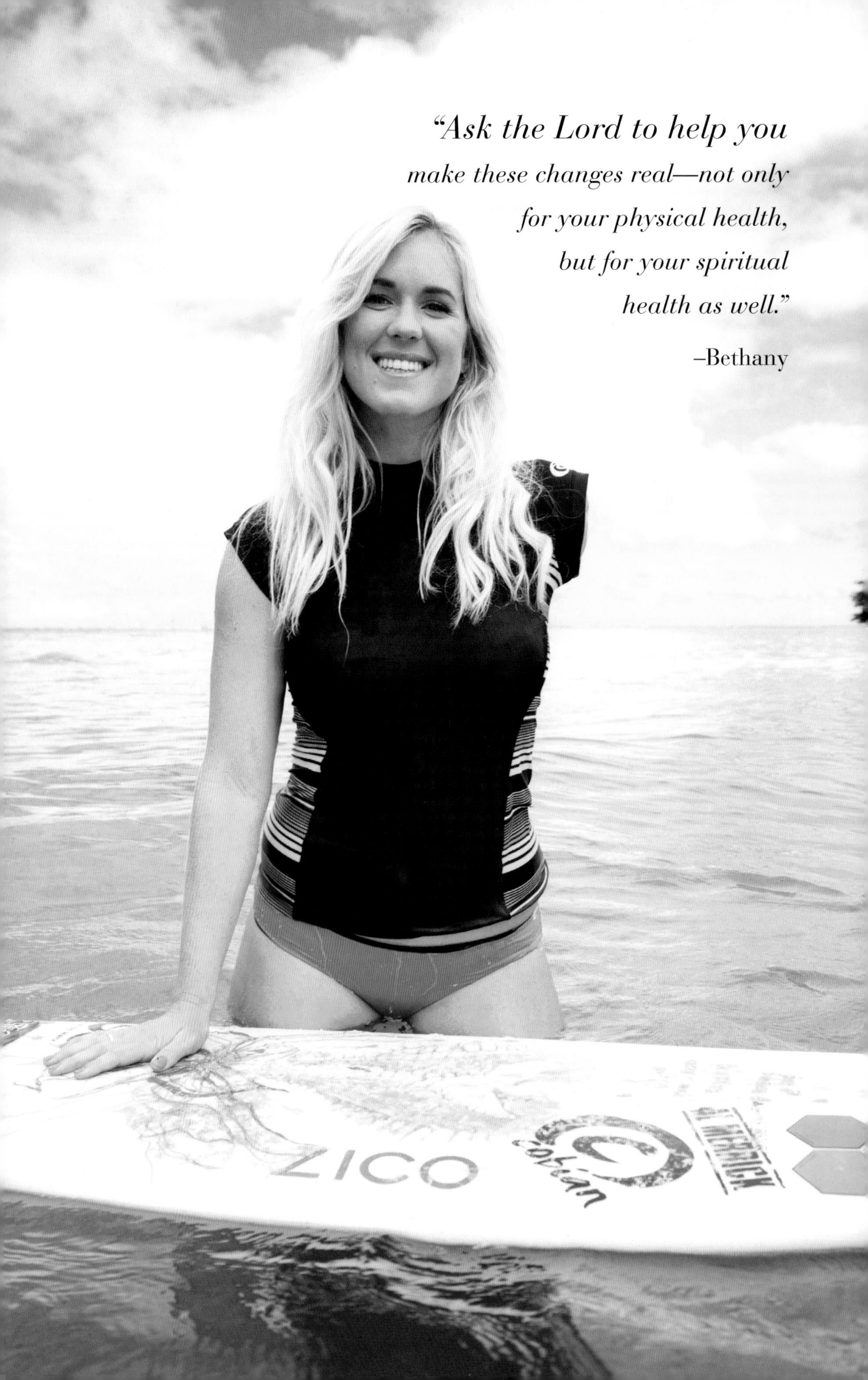
"Ask the Lord to help you make these changes real—not only for your physical health, but for your spiritual health as well."
–Bethany
ZICO

CHAPTER 6

Tackle Your Challenges

There's no place you'll get more variety than the ocean. The tides change. The waves are either awesome or "meh." Some days, the sun warms up the water to bath-like temps. Other days, it's chilly enough to wear a wetsuit.

And that's what I love so much about surfing—you really never know what you're going to get out there. Every day on my board is different and presents a new kind of challenge, which helps me learn and grow as a surfer. It's always fresh and keeps me anticipating my next surf.

Life's a lot like that too: You may think you know what's happening in your day, and then *wham!* Something happens to totally toss you out of your element. Though it can be tough to navigate change, it can be just what you need to become a stronger, smarter, and more soulful person.

That's why I'm tackling some of the common problems girls face when they start to make healthy changes. Whether you hate exercising or have fallen into the trap of doing the same workout over and over, let's burst through the Q&A's on the following pages to help you get on a happy, healthy track.

Girls Ask...

I absolutely hate the gym. I know it's good for me, but I just can't drag myself there. Any advice for what I can do instead?

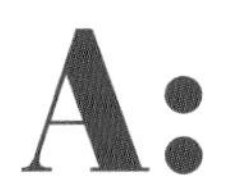

Girl, there's a whole wide world of awesome, body-blasting activities out there. While it'd be great if you loved to hit the gym daily, it's not for everyone (promise me you'll try Dustin's awesome workouts at least once). That said, if pumping iron and spending time on the treadmill aren't for you, forget it. Here are a few fun ways to break a sweat. Some require good weather or an outing but others can be done right in your backyard—or bedroom.

SO MUCH TO DO

WATER SPORTS Kayaking and canoeing are both great ways to work your arms and core, and take in awesome scenery. Supping (stand-up paddle-boarding) is a total body workout.

BARRE OR ZUMBA Love to shake it? These classes pump music while you boogie your brains out. Barre classes focus more on ballet- and Pilates-inspired moves, while Zumba is a dance party. I love to do these classes with my friends!

ROCK CLIMBING OR BOULDERING I'm not saying you need to tackle crazy canyons, but heading to a rock-climbing gym can be a cool way to test your upper-body strength—and it will be tested!

SWIMMING Some girls hang up their suits when summer is over, but in Hawaii we splash all year 'round. If swimming is your favorite, why not get a membership to a local pool so you can do laps all year long?

BIKE RIDING Your two-wheeler might be a little dusty, but hitting a bike trail with your BFFs can be really invigorating. If it's too cold, try a spinning class, where you'll pedal like mad to awesome music (and the teacher in spin class totally pumps you up!).

AERIAL YOGA If regular stretching and posing are too slow for you, consider flipping the practice upside down. Aerial yoga will have you hanging from the ceiling (literally) as you gently stretch in cool silk-like hammocks. It might sound wacky, but it's popping up in studios around the country.

TRY A MINI TRI Triathlons are major feats to undertake—unless you get a little creative. If you've got a couple hours on your hands, why not do a workout mash-up? Don't just limit yourself to running, swimming, and biking. Why not bike, jump rope, and then rollerblade? Or you could hula-hoop, run, and then do pilates.

PILATES A type of exercise that can be done on a mat or with special machines that focuses on core strength and flexibility.

EVERYTHING YOU NEED FOR A PORTABLE "GYM"

Here's all you need for a portable gym, no membership required!

- **A pair of running shoes.** You can usually go on a run no matter where you are.
- **A jump rope.** It's an excellent cardio blast you can do anywhere.
- **A yoga mat.** Loosen up your joints and get that oxygen flowing with stretches and an impromptu floor routine. (A towel works too.)

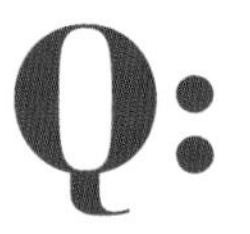

So, this is crazy to admit, but I've never really exercised regularly before. I've tried a bunch of stuff in the past, but I've never stuck with anything. Any advice to help me find my groove?

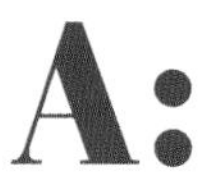

I feel blessed to have found my passion at such a young age, but it doesn't happen to everyone. Here's how to figure out if you're a cardio-burnin' babe or more of an adventure-seeking sister. Take the quiz, and then jump right in.

WHAT'S YOUR STYLE?

1. What's on your workout playlist?

A. Rap, pop, 80s—anything upbeat that gets you psyched to sweat.

B. Nothing—you like hearing the sounds of nature when you exercise. No iPod for you.

C. Electronic dance music—it really helps you get into the zone.

2. What do you like the most about running laps in gym class?

A. Beating your time from last week—and all the boys.

B. Being outside. It's so much better than being cooped up in class.

C. Getting some time to be alone with your thoughts and sort out your probs.

3. How do you know if you've gotten in a great workout?

A. You're drenched in sweat, and your heart is racing a mile a minute.

B. You've accomplished something mega like hiking a mountain or biking 20 miles.

C. You're completely clear-headed and ready to tackle your next challenge.

4. Time to sign up for extra-currics at school. What tops your list?

A. The track team. You're super competitive and love to run.

B. Nature club. If it's in the great outdoors, it's for you.

C. Yoga class. You're finally ready to master that handstand.

5. Your crush asks if you and your girls are up for a friendly game of dodgeball against his crew. Your response?

A. Game on. You can totally take him on the court.

B. Suggest you go for a bike ride instead.

C. Thanks, but no thanks. Team sports just aren't your thing.

MOSTLY A'S: MOTORIN' MAMA

Energetic and athletic, you love to get your sweat on. You'll thrive in an environment where you're challenging yourself while seeing how you stack up against the competition.

Try: High-Intensity Interval Training (HIIT), CrossFit, spinning, Tabata, Zumba.

MOSTLY B'S: GREAT OUTDOORS GIRL

A nature lover, you'd rather go for a walk in the woods than do a session on the elliptical any day. Your ideal workout involves anything that lets you breathe in the fresh air and bask in the sunshine.

Try: Trail running, cross-country skiing or snowshoeing, road or mountain biking, surfing.

MOSTLY C'S: CHILL-OUT CHICA

The hectic pace of competitive sports just isn't for you. You're happy with low-key exercises that get ya loose, lean, limber, and totally blissed out.

Try: Yoga or a stretch class, Pilates, Barre classes, ballet, swimming laps.

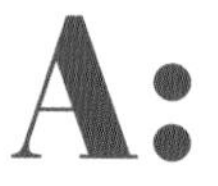

I'm trying to eat healthy, but I'm totally bored already. It's only been a week. Help?

A: First off, let me tell you, it gets easier. Over time, your body will stop craving the junk and start relishing all of God's bounty. But I know it's tough at first. Here are a few ways to make healthy eating feel more indulgent.

TIPS TO HELP YOU CRAVE HEALTHY FOODS

CRUSH YOUR CRAVINGS To beat your cravings back, trick your bod. Instead of having that huge bowl of pasta, serve up some spaghetti squash and eat it with your fave sauce. Kirby and Dustin swear by tossing everything on top of salads. If you're dying for Pad Thai, look up a recipe online and cook up the ingredients, but use just 1/3 of the noodles. Then put everything on a bed of organic shredded greens instead. The point is there are tons of ways to get all the flavors you love without all the extra junk your body doesn't need.

GO GOURMET Your school's cafeteria might not be equipped with a microwave to reheat fancy meals, but that doesn't mean your options have to be limited to the same peanut butter and jelly sandwich you always make. Ask your parents to invest in a tiffin, which is a cute stack of containers that can make lunchtime more interesting (check out happytiffin.com). You can put a stir-fry on one tier, rice on the next, and homemade pudding on the top. Or opt for soup, a salad, and a yogurt parfait.

PIECE TOGETHER A PICNIC If you and your BFFs all love to eat fantastic, fresh meals, why not team up to tackle lunch together? Once a month, work together to create an epic picnic—one person can bring greens, another can bring a bunch of crunchy toppings, someone else can bring muffins for dessert. Enlist another person to whip up a tasty juice and haul it in a canteen.

If that is too complicated, or your lunchtime is too short to enjoy it all, create a supper club where you and your friends cook together once a month. It's a great way for girls to remember that cooking isn't crazy, complicated and it helps everyone stay on track. Sleepovers don't have to be filled with chips and cookies to be a blast. My friends and I love to do Sushi night with a variety of colorful veggies, brown rice, and seared tuna. Have fun with it!

FIVE MORE WAYS TO MAKE EATING RIGHT EVEN MORE FUN

1. **START BLENDING YOUR OWN SMOOTHIES** for breakfast and snacks. Yep, it's time to open up a juice bar right in your kitchen. Getting creative with fruits, veggies, coconut water, and a blender is one way to make your after-school snack way more exciting.

2. **PARTICIPATE IN MEATLESS MONDAY.** One day a week, go veggie, along with tons of people across the country. Cooking sans meat is a speedy way to figure out just how versatile vegetables can be.

3. **FREEZE IT!** Turn fruits into cold 'n' quick snacks by tossing them into the freezer (blueberries and grapes are perfect for this), or use a combo of juice and fresh fruit to make ice pops. Yum.

4. **TEST YOUR SKILLS.** OK, so there are likely going to be times when you're really craving macaroni and cheese or a huge scoop of ice cream. While it's fine to treat yourself sometimes, get into the habit of making healthier versions of your comfort food faves. Learning to remake a classic to meet your new healthy-girl ways is one of the best parts of getting in the kitchen.

5. **SNAG ONE NEW INGREDIENT A WEEK.** I could eat apples every day, and you likely have your go-to's as well. Instead of falling in the trap of eating the same five foods—boring!—mix it up at the grocery store or farmer's market. Ask Mom to buy something new or buy one ingredient you've never tried and figure out what in the world to do with it.

I keep falling off the healthy-girl path. I know what I'm passionate about (cycling!), and I know it's important to eat better, but I just don't.

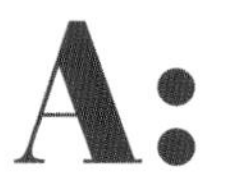

We've all been there. You read something super-inspiring and make the decision to overhaul your life all at once. As much as change can lead to amazing results, it can also be challenging. Which means if you try to undertake too many swaps at the same time, you might end up bailing on all of them.

SMALL CHANGES, BIG RESULTS

When you're just starting out, try tackling one challenge per week. The first week, aim to increase your water intake. Maybe the second week, you'll start adding some strength training to your cycling routine. The third, you could swap out your daily cookie habit for fruit, or trade your PB&J for a salad topped with chicken and avocado.

Yes, the changes are small and you might be psyched to tackle more, but going slowly through this transition will allow the changes to become a real part of your life. Soon they'll just be your new habits, and you won't even think about reaching for a plum instead of a cupcake, or going for a three-hour hike on a weekend morning. It's about creating a healthy, soulful life you love—for the long run.

Also, it's important to remember to pray about it. Ask the Lord to help you make these changes real—not only for your physical health, but for your spiritual health as well. It's actually WAY more important to be healthy spiritually and in a good relationship with God than to be consumed with physical conditioning.

Do not conform to the pattern of this world, but be transformed by the renewing of your mind.

—ROMANS 12:2

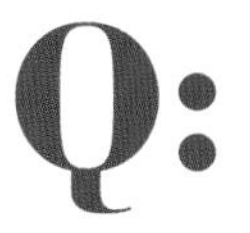

I've been able to make a lot of the changes you've suggested, but, I have to tell you, I'm not feeling that psyched about it. I was into it at first, but now I feel more like I'm going through the motions. I'm sticking with the plan, but it's just not fun for me. What's up?.

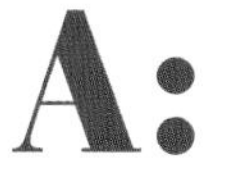

If you're super busy and keeping a million balls in the air, but not enjoying anything, you might be headed toward burnout. It's actually great that you noticed it now, before you got sick, injured, or just totally gave up. Here are a few ways to know if you're about to burn out ... and what to do about it.

SIGNS YOU MAY BE BURNED OUT

1. **YOU'RE TOTALLY TIRED.** I'm not just talking about getting sleepy during your fifth-period bio class. If you're exhausted from the time you wake up to the time you go to bed, it's a sure sign you're doing too much.
2. **YOU'RE SNAPPY.** You argue with your parents, constantly bicker with your sibs, and can't seem to get along with your crew. The stress you're under can cause your patience to wear thin, making you easily frustrated and annoyed with others.
3. **YOU'RE FORGETFUL.** With so much on your plate, it's getting impossible to keep track of every last detail. The result? You're more absent-minded than ever, causing you to miss out on some pretty important stuff.
4. **YOU'RE INDIFFERENT.** You used to feel absolutely amazing when you got an A on a test or scored the most points in your volleyball game. Now? Not so much. If you're lacking enthusiasm for something you were once really excited about, it's probably time to step away so you can reignite that passion.
5. **YOU'RE OVERWHELMED.** Here's the clincher: whenever you take on more than you can handle, it's virtually inevitable that you'll crash and, well, burn out. If you constantly feel like there's just not enough time to get everything done, then there probably isn't.

IF YOU ARE HEADED TOWARDS BURNOUT

Don't stress. The first step is recognizing that you need to make a change. Carve out some time to reassess what you need to do—whether it's dropping an extra-curric or sharing your soccer captain duties with a teammate. Bottom line: Do what's best for you in the bigger picture, don't be afraid to say no to something, and don't be afraid to ask for help whenever you need it. Before you know it, you'll be back on track, refreshed and refocused.

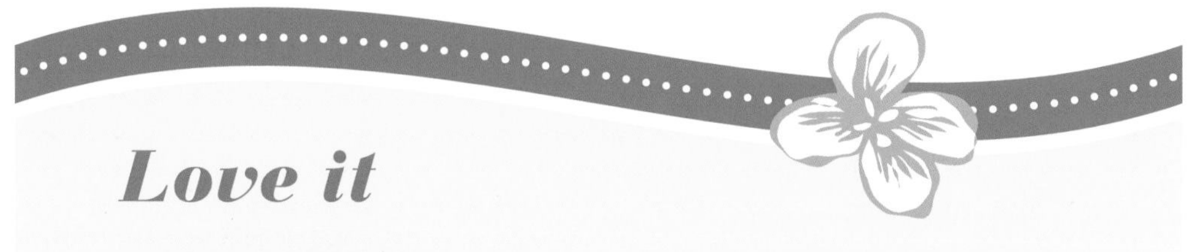

Love it

* **JUST ONCE** Saying "just once" and indulging yourself is good to reduce burnout and feelings of deprivation, and allowing yourself a treat now and then will help you stay on track. But don't let "just once" turn into lots and lots of "just once's."
* **BALANCE** You need it when it comes to your meals, workout routines, sleep, and time with family, friends, and God.
* **CONSISTENCY** Don't work your butt off for a week and just stop after that. The more you keep things up, the easier it is to stay on track.

Dump it

* **FAT FREE** Fat free does not mean better. Food processors may remove some fat, but it's replaced with chemicals. Check food labels.
* **DIET** Be wary of the word *diet*. Diet can make you feel self-deprived. Instead think healthy.
* **BUSY** There's always time to take care of your health.

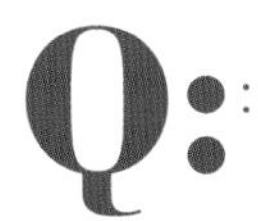

My friends and I want to exercise together, but we always just end up sitting around, not really sure what to do. Advice, please.

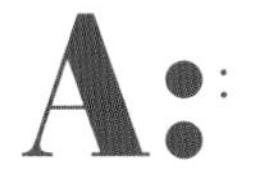

There's nothing worse than thinking you and your BFFs are gonna get a great workout in, and then you just end up going for a half-hearted jog. I love playing soccer, hiking, biking, roller blading, swimming, and playing tennis and even stretching with my crew. When I'm having a blast with my buds, I don't even notice that I'm sweating buckets on a hike or have been whacking a tennis ball for hours. It definitely puts the play back in your workout.

To make it an effective workout, though, you're going to need some structure. Otherwise, you will spend more time chatting than sweating. Here are a few tips for making the most of your time together.

Work in tandem while you're at the gym. Don't love strength training? Find a bud who does, and alternate reps with her. She'll do her squats while you count, and then you switch, keeping each other accountable for each and every exercise. Make sure to blast the music to keep the tempo up.

Sign up for a race together. Whether there's a charity you want to support or a mud run you're dying to do, having a goal on the horizon is bound to keep you and your BFF on track. Write down your training plan to make it concrete.

Tackle a twosome task. You might feel a little goofy, but taking a partner to yoga class, riding a tandem bike, or getting into a two-girl kayak are all ways to boost your friendship and ensure that each girl is pulling her own weight. Or create a challenge for yourselves: plan to run the stairs at the local football stadium or do a tough Pilates YouTube video in your living room.

Take the hardest class at the gym (to you!). Sometimes when friends exercise together, they fall into super cinchy routines, walking the same route again and again. Break the pattern by challenging yourselves to take the class at your local Y that scares you the most, whether that's karate, volleyball, or beginner's ballet. Being on a schedule will ensure you two are sweating at regular intervals—together.

Q: I've been getting sooo bored during my workouts. Ugh. I just end up spacing out. If I have to do another lunge, I might cry!

A: Not only is spacing out a sign that your workout isn't interesting enough, it's downright dangerous (hello, you could get hurt). Luckily, there are plenty of ways to get some pep back in your step.

Get goofy. Try creating a wacky cardio routine that corresponds to an upbeat playlist: Assign each song an exercise, like a sprint or a set of jumping jacks or surfer burpees (see page 74). Then put your iPod on shuffle and do at least thirty seconds of each move. Trust me, you'll be zonked—and it's like having a personal DJ at your house.

Reconfigure your sweat sesh. If you're always doing the same old, same old, it's bound to get boring. That said, you can't abandon the basics. What's a girl to do? Infuse some life into your strength routine by adding a cardio burst (do two sets of moves, then take a lap around the gym). On a long run or cardio session? Give yourself mini missions along the way: I'll make it to that lamppost in twenty seconds. Or sprint to that mailbox. When I get to that mailbox, I'll do a set of high knees. Keep your brain on its toes to stay interested in what you're doing.

Do a body or breath check. When you're on a long run or hike or swim, it can be easy to zone out. Instead of turning into a space case, stay present by checking in on your body every few minutes. Do a full-body scan to see how you feel. Then spend a few cycles paying attention to your breath. Is it slow and smooth, or fast and jagged? Attempting to even it out can make you feel better out there. Then repeat.

Be proud—then push yourself. OK, so if you're headed to another planet while you're working out, you're probably not challenging yourself at all. Take a sec to congratulate yourself for how far you've come, then know it's time to crank it once more. Whether you need to add more reps, more weights, more distance or more variety, make the change and then go for it—again.

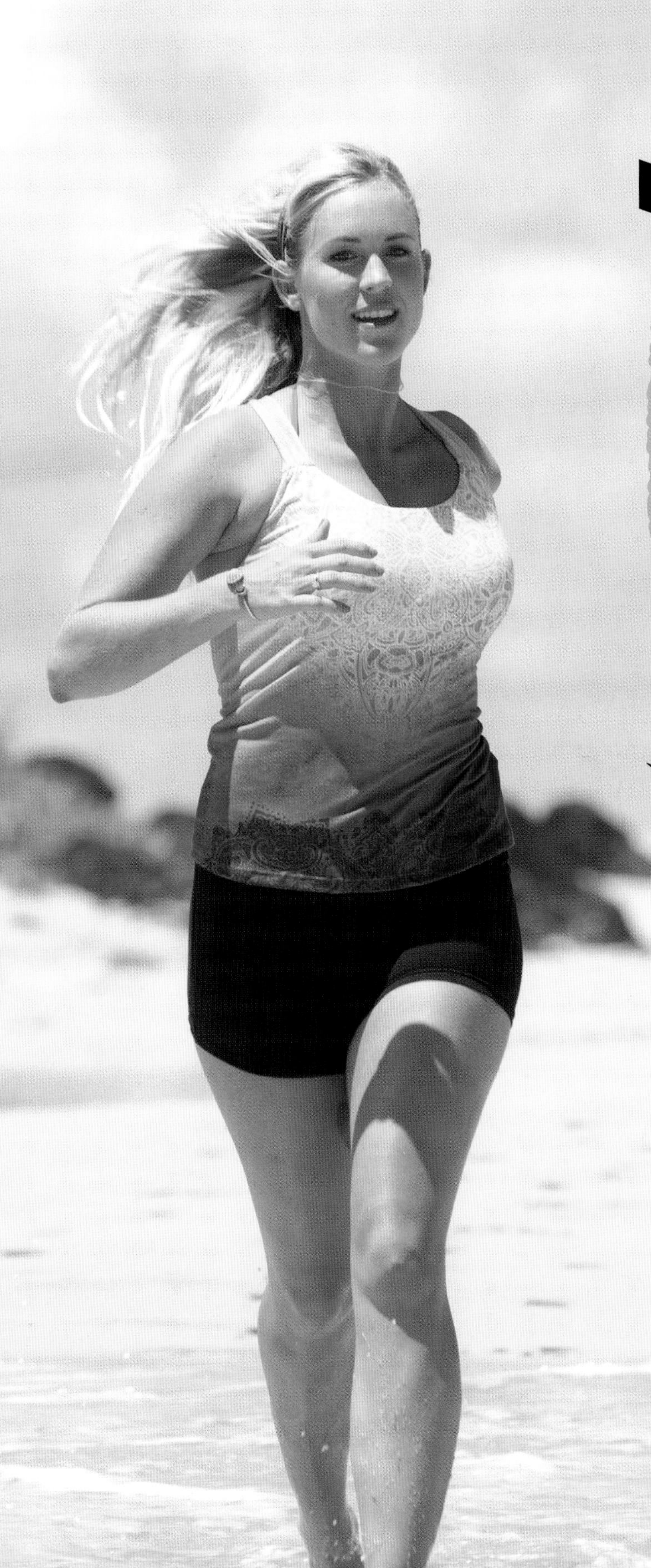

BETHANY'S SOUL SECRET

One of my favorite trainers once encouraged me to work hard and "rest as much as you play."

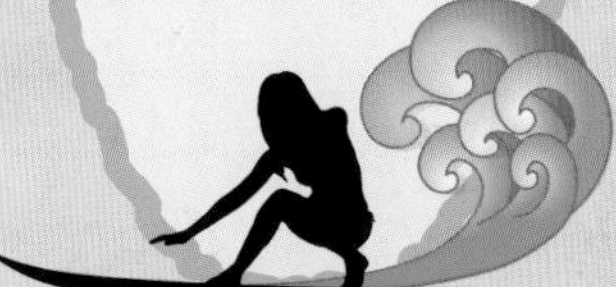

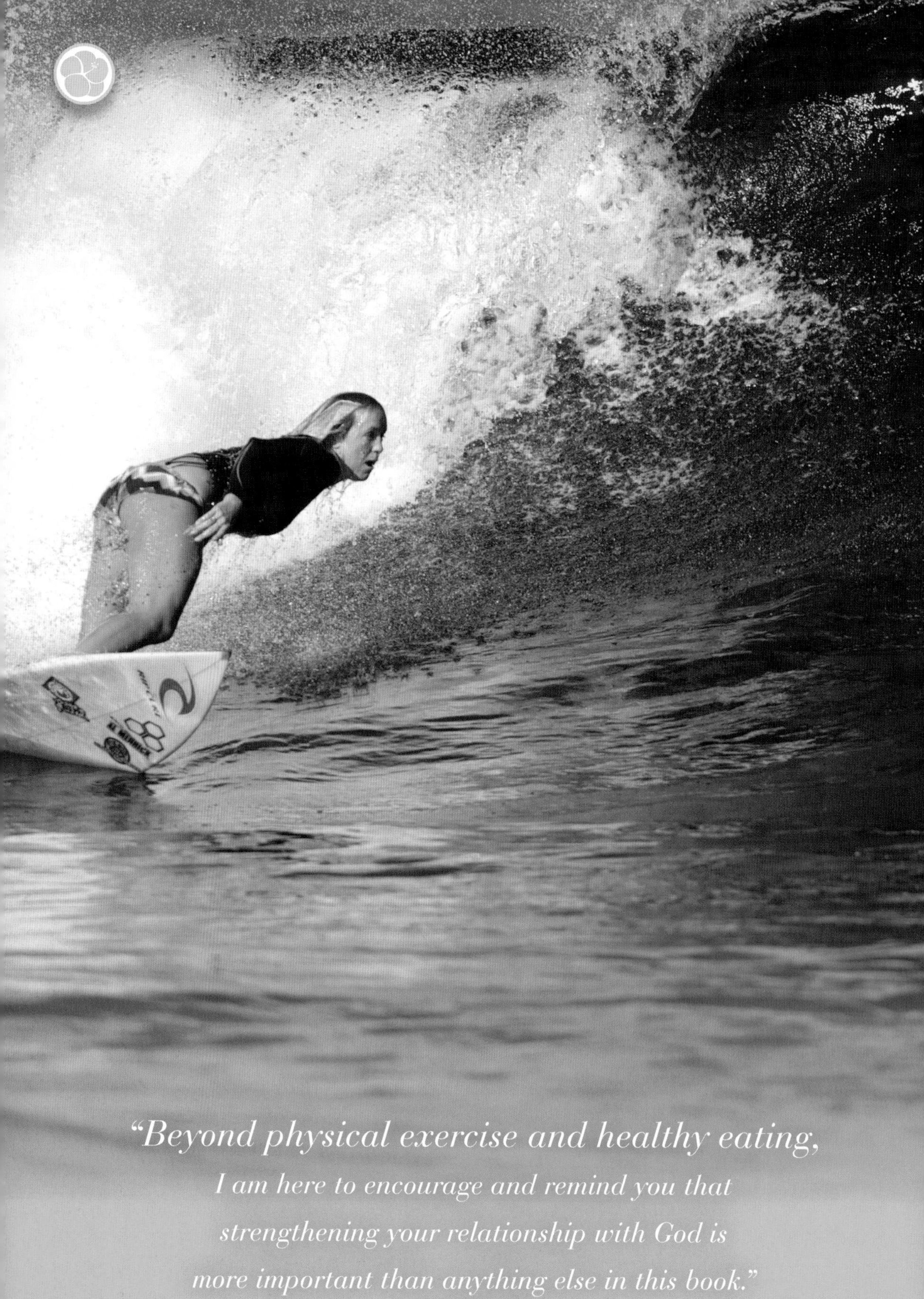

"Beyond physical exercise and healthy eating,
I am here to encourage and remind you that
strengthening your relationship with God is
more important than anything else in this book."
—Bethany

CHAPTER 7

Go the Distance

For physical training is of some value, but godliness has value for all things, holding promise for both the present life and the life to come.

—1 TIMOTHY 4:8

The Bible notes there is value in taking care of your physical body. I promise, if you incorporate exercise and healthy eating into your life, you can accomplish much more throughout your day and feel better about yourself. But beyond physical exercise and healthy eating, I am here to encourage and remind you that strengthening your relationship with God is more important than anything else in this book.

Take my shark attack, for example. Do you think I saw that coming? God took what seemed like a tragedy and turned it into something beautiful. I may be missing my left arm, but I still have my life! I have been able to keep doing the things I love, and I have been able to see God work through my life. He has taken me to experience amazing opportunities I may never have known if I hadn't trusted in him during my incident. And better yet, I've been able to share the love of God with others!

I've gone from a young girl just doing an activity her whole family enjoys, to landing a dozen top ten placements in Association of Surfing Professionals and World Tour Events (the major leagues of surfing). I've surfed the warm, powerful water of Indonesia, enjoyed time in Nicaragua, and even caught some fun waves in Australia.

I'm surfing with only one arm, with the top women surfers in the world, and I'm rockin' it!

Life happens. Stuff gets in the way. You have to learn to trust in God through setbacks. They often aren't in your control; and that's OK. We shouldn't be "in control" God should. Putting your trust in God in all things will help you in your journey—in getting fit and in all aspects of your life. Every time we put our trust in God, I picture us bringing a huge smile to his face.

I consider my relationship with God the most important relationship in my life. How do I nurture my relationship with him? By spending time with God in prayer and reading his Word, the Bible, listening, and obeying.

If you took a look at my travel Bible right now, you'd see how thrashed it is because I take it with me wherever I go. I encourage you to "thrash your Bible," dig into God's Word, be intentional in your reading, and ask God to have the Holy Spirit reveal to you the areas in your life he wants to work on. It really is cool when God reveals to us those areas in our life. A lot of times it's challenging to face our sin, but it really is a good thing—his discipline is given to bring us closer to him. Having a relationship with Jesus Christ will help put things into perspective and show you what's truly important in your life. I really do think that we become what we focus on. So if you focus on living out your life for God and others, it will be hard not to succeed.

NURTURE THE LOVE AROUND YOU

In the same way, it's important to nurture all the relationships in your life—your family and friends and all those God brings into your life.

If you think about it, nurturing your relationships is just as vital as nurturing your body. Even more so, it's the second greatest commandment—"love your neighbor." Personal relationships are your foundation. It's important to have people in your life who will give you encouragement throughout your life. So I encourage you to be intentional in the way you approach your relationships. You too can be loving and help others no matter how young you are; you can be an encouraging example too!

Let no one despise you for your youth, but set the believers an example in speech, in conduct, in love, in faith, in purity.

—1 TIMOTHY 4:12 ESV

Staying balanced is a great way to become more grounded and keep connected to those around you. Someone recently painted a word picture for me on the subject. Say you're walking around carrying a bunch of plates. All the plates have food on them. But if you start putting more on only one plate, all the others are going to come crashing down.

I love that picture because I have a lot of plates—there's surfing, doing well in competition, working with my sponsors, motivational speaking, staying healthy and fit, finding time to rest, making good choices, nurturing my relationships, and deepening my faith. Whatever your desires are, finding balance is really important.

When I'm traveling, I always remember to email my family pictures of my adventures. And when I get back, we carve out time to have a barbecue or I'll surf with my bros. After being apart from my friends, we'll hang out or go to a fun workout class like a Zumba session or a crossfit style workout class. It's a great way to bond. And when it's over, instead, we talk about how we felt during the workout. Did we feel strong that time? Did it push our limits? And the next day we'll share with each other how sore our muscles are!

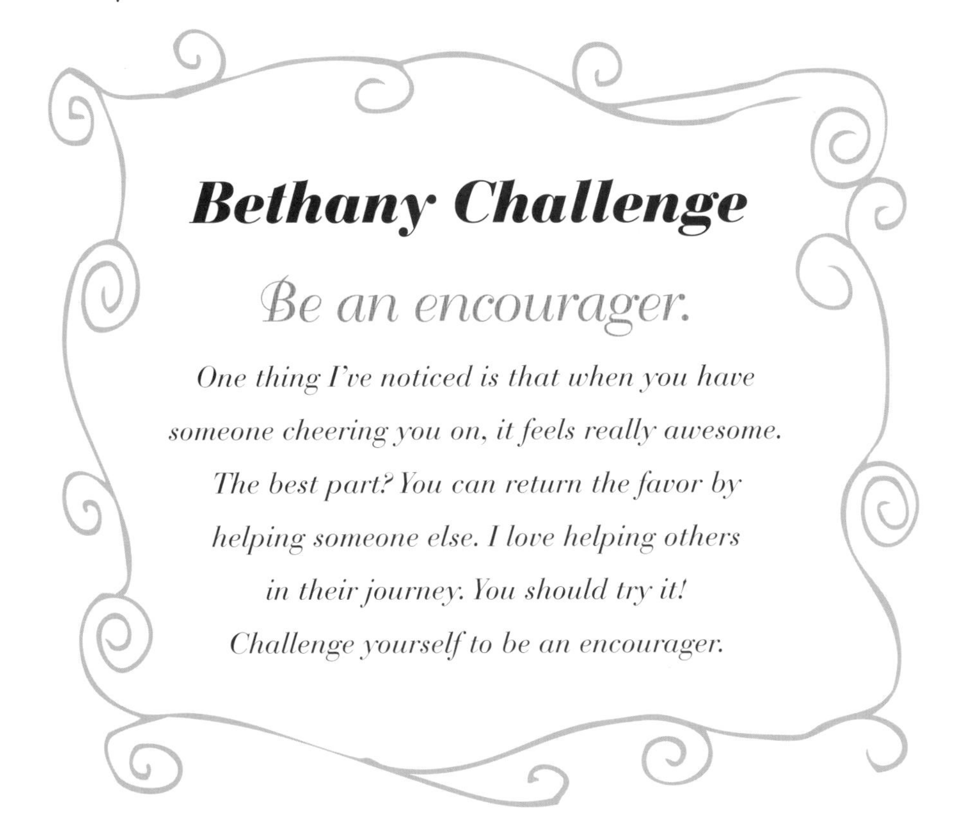

Bethany Challenge

Be an encourager.

One thing I've noticed is that when you have someone cheering you on, it feels really awesome. The best part? You can return the favor by helping someone else. I love helping others in their journey. You should try it! Challenge yourself to be an encourager.

Do you not know that in a race all the runners run, but only one gets the prize? Run in such a way as to get the prize.
1 CORINTHIANS 9:24

So maybe after all you've read, you've made a commitment to improve your eating and fitness regimen. Right on! Don't give up if you can't see results right away. You might not like the new green additions to your diet for a couple weeks, and you might not gain confidence from seeing your body get stronger until next month. Just give everything a decent chance.

How do you make sure you stay on course? By never losing sight of your goals. By knowing what you believe in and what you hope to achieve. And by seeing the ways your life improves over time with the changes you make.

BETHANY'S SOUL SECRET

Having a buddy system helps. My hubby pushes me. Grab a friend or family member and push each other!

Try setting short-term goals. Say your goal is to lose five pounds. Within that goal, you might make a plan to run ten miles in a week. So you divide that up and plan to run two miles a day for five days.

Or you may set a goal of holding a plank for one minute, but starting out you can only hold for twenty seconds. Make a goal to practice your plank every day, and add ten seconds each day. Work hard and gradually build yourself up to that point—short-term plans are the way to go. Set goals that are obtainable, and you will be setting yourself up for success and more positive results later—you have to be patient with the process.

For me, I have a hard time running. Going for a jog doesn't come naturally for me. But I keep doing it and know that I'll reach my goal to run farther eventually.

Once you reach a goal, continue to challenge yourself by setting new goals. Whether I'm surfing in a heat or going out just for fun, I always want to surf my best. I like to push myself and find ways to get better and better.

You just hit eight laps in the pool? Challenge yourself to do two extra the next go-around. Finding new ways to trump your personal bests will keep your passion and drive alive for as long as you will allow, giving you a sense of fulfillment while keeping the possibilities open for new achievements.

And, obviously, you're entitled to a break sometimes—and don't always be so hard on yourself. It's OK to have a cheat day, and it's fine if you didn't get through your planned workout set last week. Just start again the next day.

Therefore, since we are surrounded by such a great cloud of witnesses, let us throw off everything that hinders and the sin that so easily entangles. And let us run with perseverance the race marked out for us.

—HEBREWS 12:1

Perseverance is something that takes practice—both in the physical sense and in your spiritual life. Physically we may have obstacles that hinder or entangle us while on the way to our goals, and it's the same in your journey with God. This verse from Hebrews 12 encourages us to stop participating in things that distract us from our goals and what God wants for our lives.

We all have different personalities and different lifestyles. Maybe you're balancing school with your booming weekend babysitting business. Maybe you signed up for too many activities, and all your days are starting to blur together. I encourage you to not let your busy schedule be an excuse to skip a workout session or opt for the quicker and easier fast food choice. Figuring out how to be consistent with your fitness and diet plans, no matter the circumstances, will help you establish healthy habits for life.

You probably shouldn't go into every situation expecting you'll be the winner every time. It takes time to learn and get better at things. In the big picture—especially in the beginning of your journey—it's about going into your situation with the right attitude and about being a good team player, or being adventurous and push yourself to try things you normally wouldn't attempt.

BETHANY'S SOUL SECRET

I've noticed with fitness and nutrition, when you don't keep up, it's hard to get back into it. When you lose your momentum, you're gonna have a hard time getting yourself back into the routine.

If you're discouraged, give it to God. I recommend praying every day for endurance, wisdom, and self-control. Ask God for help in the areas that may be a struggle. Having strong faith enables you to have a sense of peace, even when everything around you seems daunting. Just be patient as you strive to reach your goals.

Part of being patient includes being flexible. Say it's raining outside and you were supposed to go on a run with your friends. Instead of moping, turn it into another awesome activity. Maybe stay inside and try some new healthy recipes—and have a dance party while doing it! There are always active, healthy things you can be doing no matter the circumstances.

Do nothing out of selfish ambition or vain conceit. Rather, in humility value others above yourselves, not looking to your own interests but each of you to the interests of others. In your relationships with one another, have the same mindset as Christ Jesus.

—PHILIPPIANS 2:3-5

With all your exercising and eating right, you'll be so confident and stoked, it will be easy to brag about it and want *everyone* to go on this journey with you. But remember not everyone is ready or able to do that. Instead, just encourage your friends and family to try a new workout move or a delicious new dish.

I'm all for the theory of striving to do your best, but in a humble way. Ask others about their goals or achievements. The bottom line? Your aim should just be to motivate and encourage each other. And while you are lifting up the people around you, remember there's always room for you to grow too.

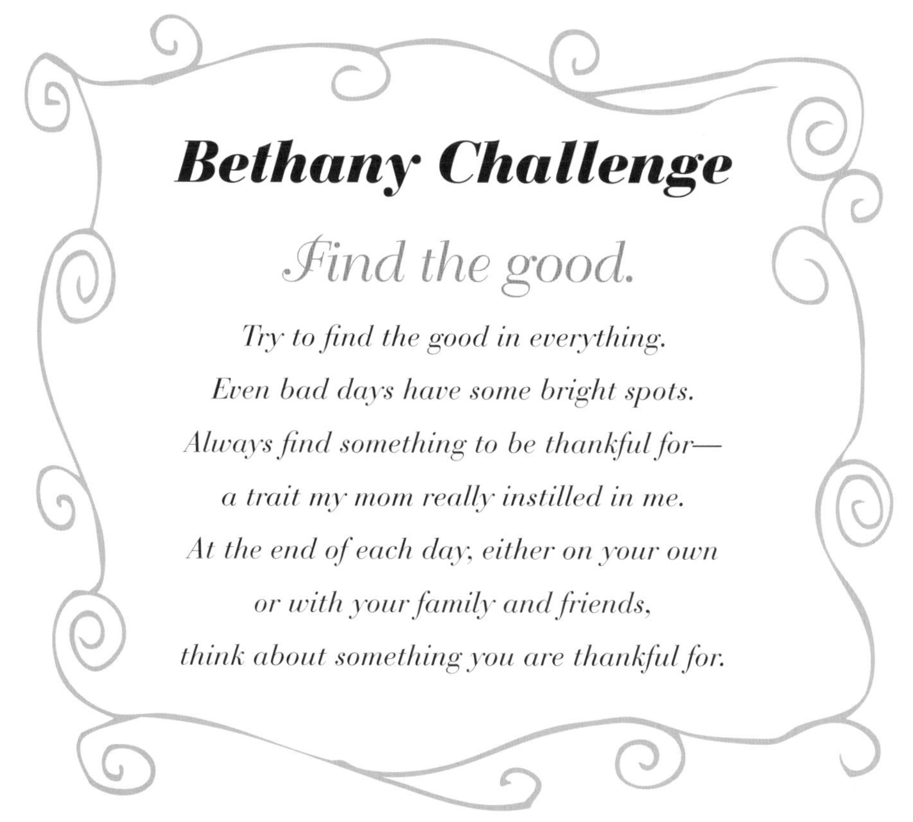

Bethany Challenge

Find the good.

Try to find the good in everything.
Even bad days have some bright spots.
Always find something to be thankful for—
a trait my mom really instilled in me.
At the end of each day, either on your own
or with your family and friends,
think about something you are thankful for.

I love working hard at whatever I attempt—and working hard to maintain a nutritious, soulful life is no exception. I am here to tell you that anyone can become just as committed to maintaining a healthy lifestyle as I have over the years.

The feeling I get when I work out, the improvements I've seen in my athletic performance, and the endurance and confidence I've gained through my journey is enough to drive me to keep it all up.

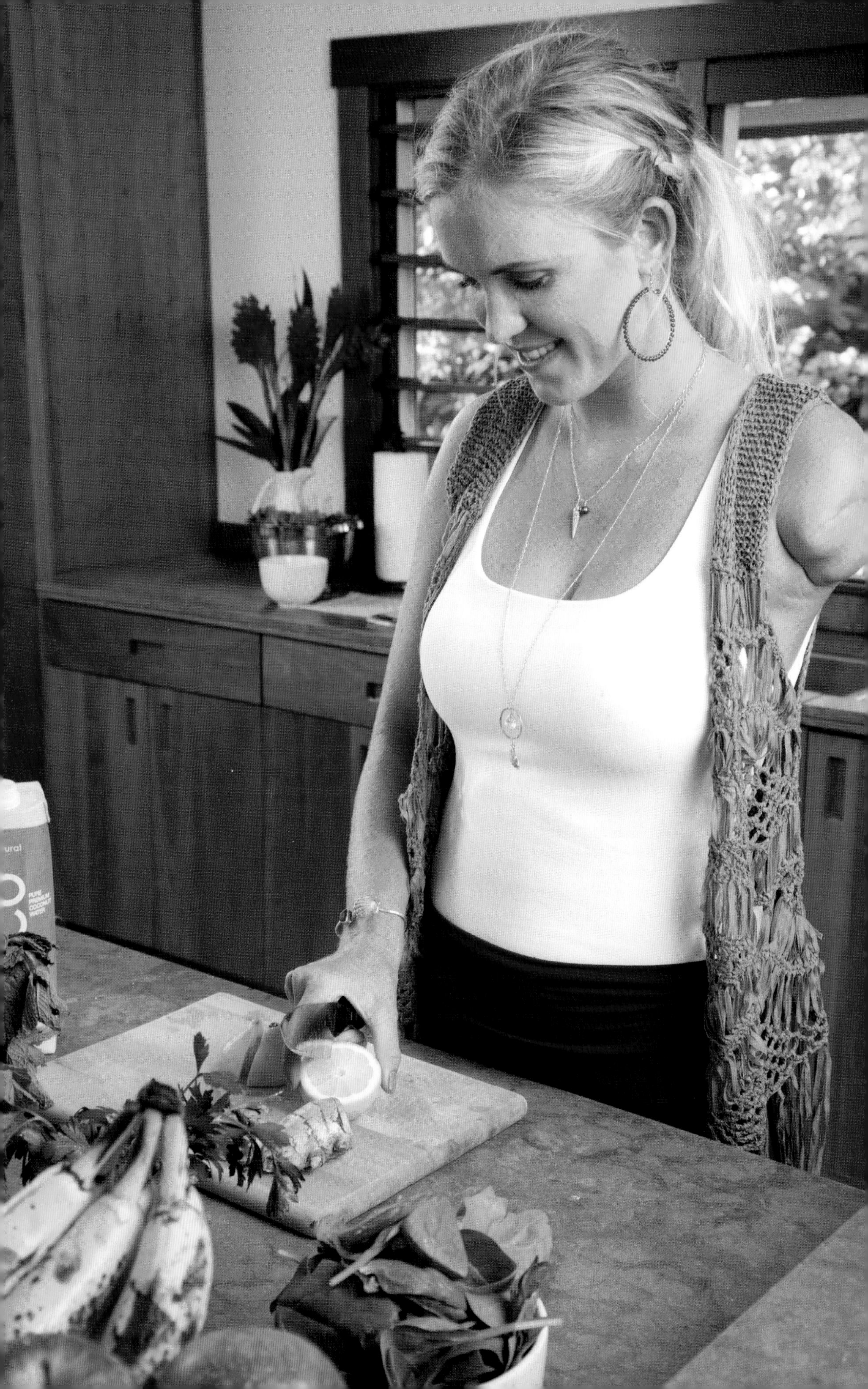
PURE
PREMIUM
COCONUT
WATER

CHAPTER 8

Clean Green Recipes

No matter where I find myself throughout the year, I'm always keeping an open mind and picking up ideas that will spice up my healthy lifestyle.

I've scored some delicious recipes from Tahiti, including an amazing coconut garlic fish dish (page 120). And even when I'm not on the road, I try to expand my cultural palate by cooking with friends. I have a friend who is Peruvian, and I love going over to her house to sample her tasty, amazing fried "rice" dish, made with quinoa (page 135). It's sooo good.

Get ready to rock your kitchen. Kirby has whipped up more than thirty easy, fun-to-make recipes for breakfast, lunch, and dinner (and everything in between). Naturally, these DIYs are super healthy and feature the freshest foods you can imagine.

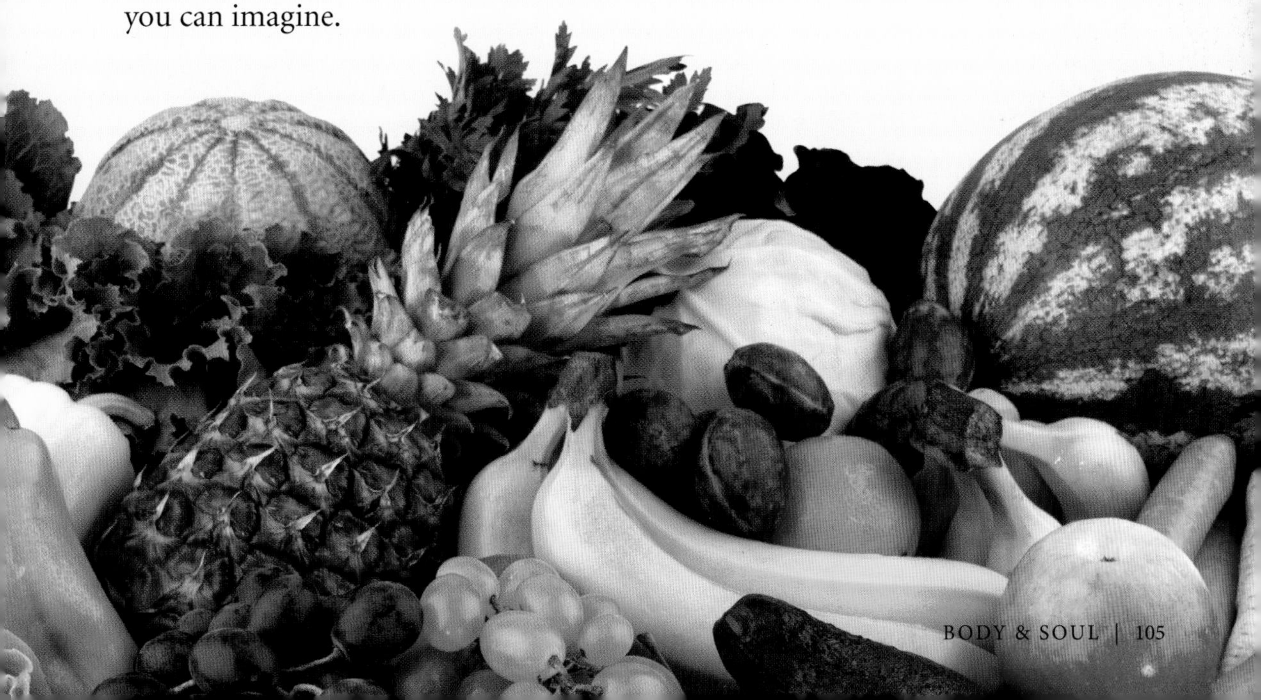

Breakfast

It's time to strike sugar-filled cereals from your morning must-have list. Whether you like to go sweet or savory in the a.m., these bites will give your body the boost it needs to get the day going.

QUINOA MORNING BOWL

Make a comforting breakfast by cooking up some quinoa at night, then top it with nuts and fruit.

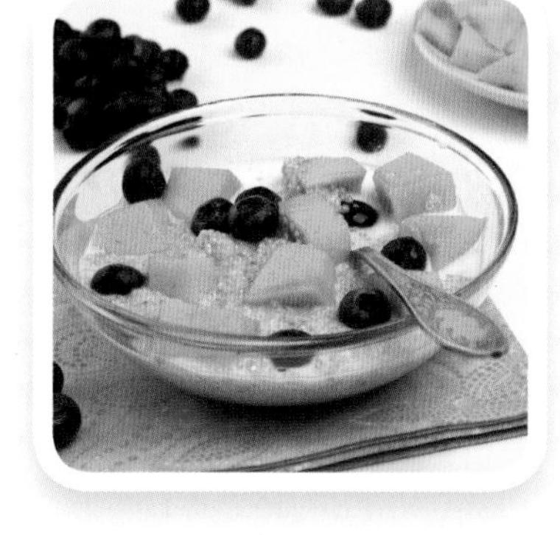

SERVES 1

1/2 cup quinoa (find it in the grain aisle)

2 tbsp. almond milk (or coconut milk)

1 tbsp. almond butter

1 tsp. grade B real maple syrup or organic honey (check the label)

1/2 banana, sliced (or your fave fruit; strawberries, blueberries, blackberries, mangoes or raspberries are all great)

Optional: cinnamon to taste, a handful of nuts — I love walnuts and almonds!

The night before you want a warm, filling breakfast, cook the quinoa by following the instructions on the package. (You might want to cook more and eat it for a couple of mornings!)

The next morning, put the quinoa, milk, almond butter, and maple syrup in a small saucepan. Reheat on medium-low, stirring, so the quinoa doesn't stick. When the mixture is warm (it should only take a few minutes), scoop it into a bowl and add the fruit and nuts.

MANGO MUFFINS

The tropics come straight to your house with these tasty treats. They contain coconut flour, which is better for you than the standard stuff and available at health food stores or online.

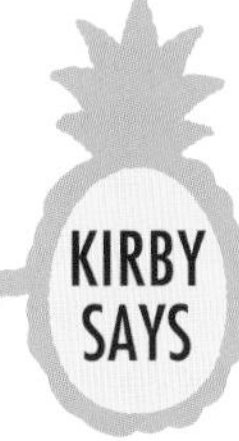

Check with your parents to see if they have a sifter, which helps get air into the flour (it can settle on the shelf). If you don't have one, no worries. Simply put a portion of flour in a bowl and whisk it. Then measure the flour.

MAKES 12 MUFFINS

1/2 cup coconut flour, sifted

1/2 tsp. sea salt

1/2 tsp. baking soda

6 organic eggs

1/3 cup grade B real maple syrup (check the label)

1/3 cup coconut oil

1 tsp. vanilla extract

1 cup diced mango, fresh or frozen

Heat oven to 350°F and line a muffin tin with paper liners. In a small bowl, combine coconut flour, salt, and baking soda. In a large bowl, combine eggs, maple syrup, coconut oil, and vanilla. Blend well with a hand mixer. Mix dry ingredients into wet; blend well. Gently fold in mango. Spoon batter into muffin cups. Bake for 20 to 25 minutes. Cool and serve.

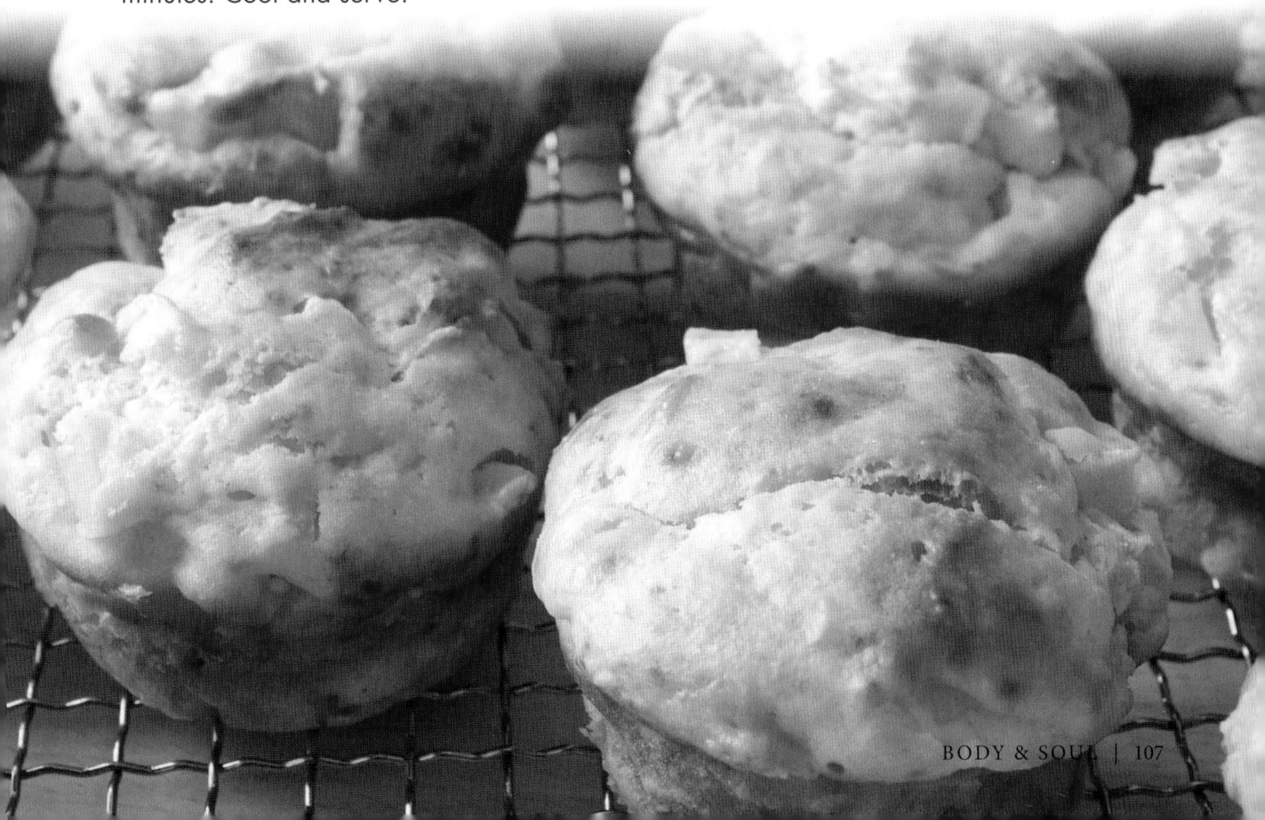

SCRAMBLED EGGS WITH PAN-ROASTED TOMATOES, GOAT CHEESE, AND FRESH BASIL

This recipe seems fancy but is a cinch to make. Brunch, anyone? I love starting my day with a nice scramble!

SERVES 2

4 large organic, free-range eggs

2 tbsp. fresh basil, coarsely chopped

Freshly ground black pepper (to taste)

2 tbsp. coconut oil

1 tbsp. shallots or onions, minced (cut into tiny pieces)

1 cup tear-drop tomatoes or baby heirloom tomatoes, sliced in half

1 tbsp. unsalted butter (grass-fed butter is best)

1/4 cup goat cheese

In a large bowl, whisk together eggs, one tablespoon basil, and black pepper. Set aside. In a large frying pan, heat coconut oil over medium heat. Add shallots and sauté, stirring occasionally for one minute or until softened. Add tomatoes and cook for one to two minutes or until they begin to soften. Place tomato mixture in bowl and set aside.

In the same pan you used for the tomatoes, melt butter over medium heat. Pour in the egg mixture and reduce the heat to medium-low. Cook the eggs until they begin to set. Stir the eggs, scrape the sides and bottom of the pan. Fold the eggs back into the center. Cook until the eggs are done (they won't be jiggly) but still moist. Add cheese and stir. Remove the pan from the heat and let stand as the cheese continues to melt. Gently fold the tomatoes into the eggs, and garnish with one tablespoon of basil.

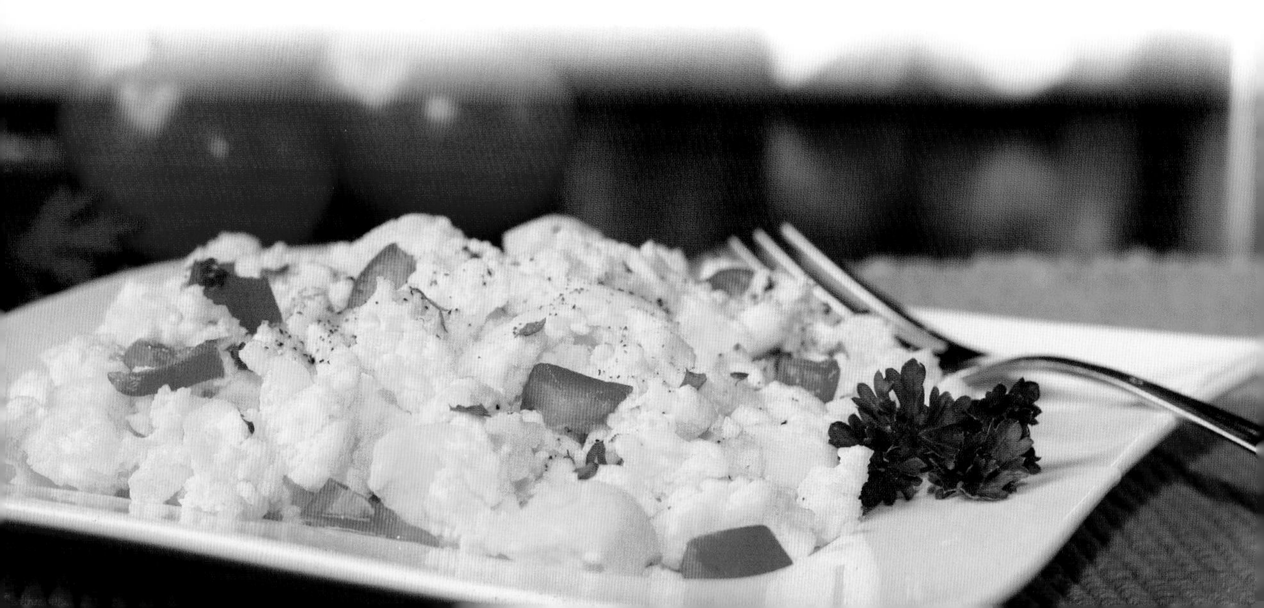

BAKED EGG AND KALE CUPS

These cute cups are fab when you're feeding your BFFs after a sleepover. Put one girl on egg duty, and stick another in charge of blending juice. Way better than a doughnut run—seriously.

SERVES UP TO 6

Olive or coconut oil, for greasing pan

Kale (1 large leaf per serving)

Eggs (1 per "cup")

Salt

Freshly ground pepper

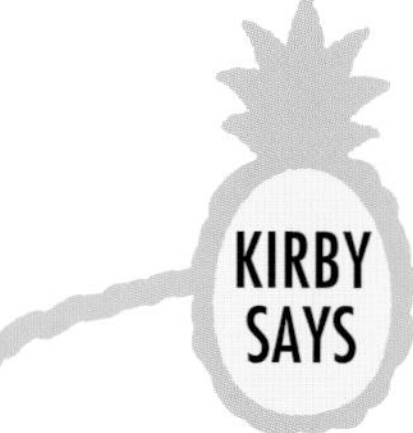

Try adding red bell peppers, onions, mushrooms, and/or zucchini in any of the egg dishes.

Heat oven to 375°F. Grease muffin tin, place on baking sheet, and set aside. Wash and trim kale, removing thick stems in the middle. Fill medium saucepan with one to two cups water and heat on medium-high. When almost boiling (bubbling, but not with big bubbles), add kale leaves and cover. Reduce heat and simmer for four to five minutes. Carefully remove leaves with slotted spoon; rinse with cool water and pat dry with a clean towel.

Line cups of prepped muffin tin with leaves of cooked kale, making sure to cover as much of the muffin cups as possible. Leave a bit of kale sticking up above the surface of the muffin tin. You'll need one large leaf per cup, but it's OK to layer several smaller leaves.

Crack one egg into each muffin cup, covering kale. Sprinkle eggs with salt and pepper. Bake for 17 to 25 minutes, until the egg yolk is set (no longer liquid). Use oven mitts to remove muffin tray from oven. Allow to cool for five minutes before carefully popping out the egg cups. Serve warm.

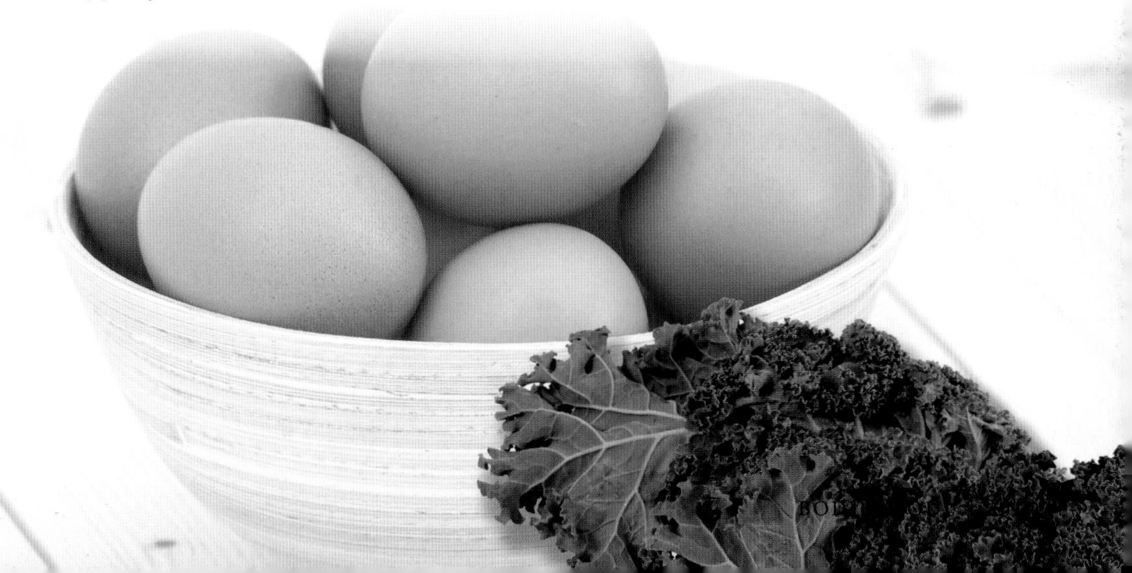

POACHED EGGS WITH KALE

Never poached an egg before? No worries. It's not as tricky as it seems—and the eggs are nice and light when they're done. We've listed this as a breakfast recipe, but it'd be perfect for lunch too.

SERVES 1

3 to 4 tbsp. white vinegar

1 organic egg

Handful baby kale leaves, washed

Coconut oil (optional)

Sea salt

Freshly ground pepper to taste

KIRBY SAYS

If you are getting tired of kale or having a tough time keeping it available in the house, mix it up. You can use other greens and veggies.

Bring a small saucepan of water to boil. Add a big splash (three to four tbsp) of white vinegar and reduce heat to a rapid simmer. Break eggs into a small bowl and slide each into the water. Simmer gently for three minutes or until cooked to your liking. Meanwhile, place kale on a serving plate. Remove eggs from the water with a slotted spoon and pat dry with a clean tea towel. Serve eggs on top of the kale seasoned with sea salt and black pepper.

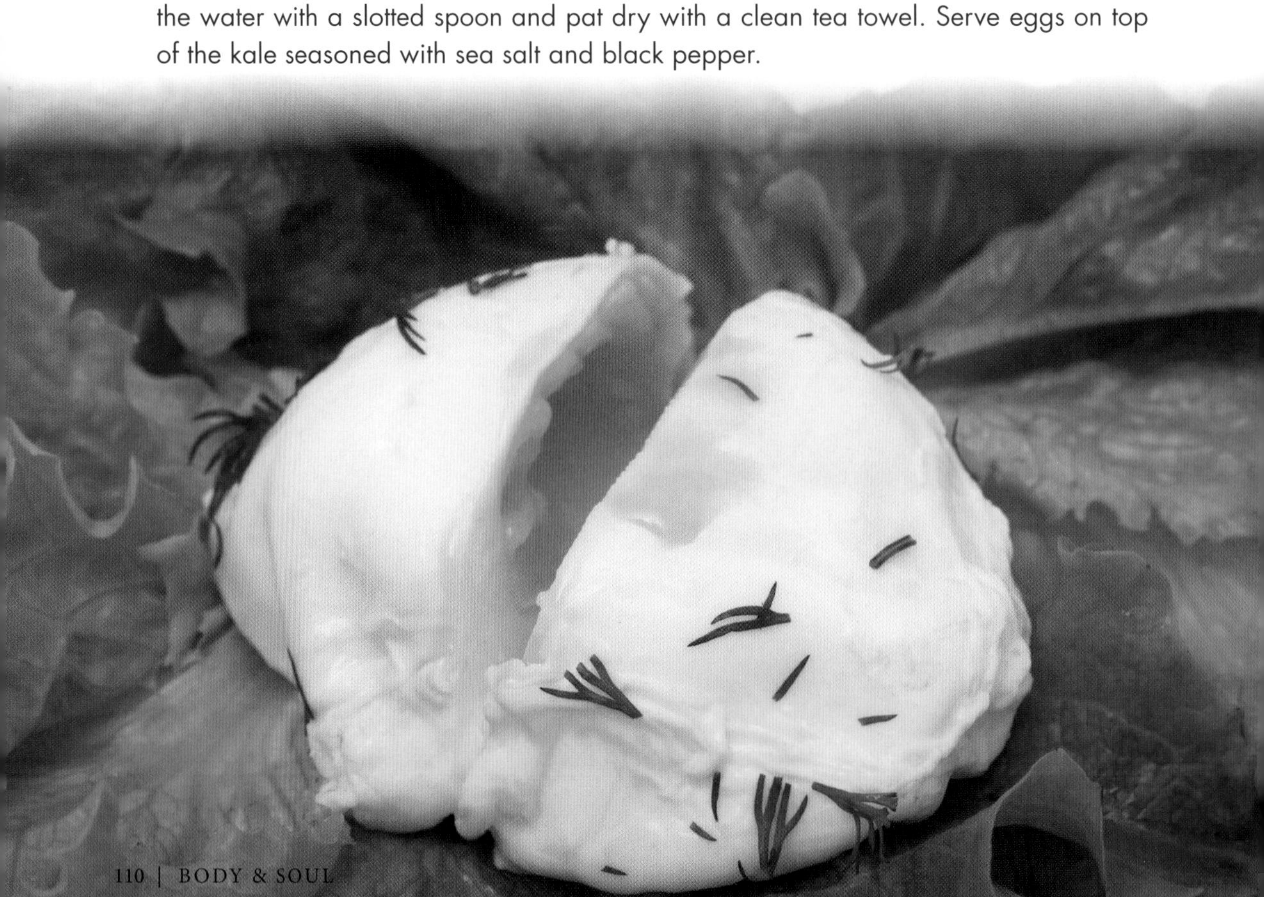

INSIDE-OUT EGGS

Don't be afraid to make eggs on school days. A hearty, veggie-filled breakfast is just what you need to get through a busy day.

SERVES 2

2 tsp. coconut oil or extra virgin olive oil

4 organic eggs

1/2 cup fresh spinach leaves or kale

2 tbsp. red bell pepper, chopped

1 tbsp. red onion, chopped

2 grape or cherry tomatoes, quartered

1 pinch salt

1 pinch pepper

1 pinch red pepper flakes (optional)

1/2 avocado cubed

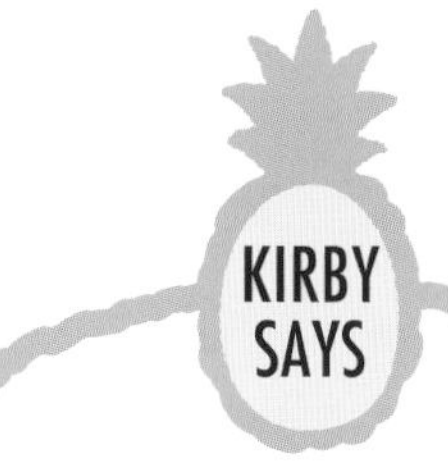

Get creative!
Throw in your favorite veggies and flavors to make this your own!

Put a medium frying pan on the stove and add oil. Heat pan with oil to medium. Add spinach or kale, bell pepper, onion, tomatoes, salt, pepper, and pepper flakes into pan. Sauté veggies until softened.

Crack eggs into a bowl and whisk to mix. Add whisked egg mixture over veggies in hot pan. Carefully slide the pan back and forth until eggs set (get firm). Right before the eggs set, drop avocado cubes in. Use a spatula to fold the omelet in half and cook for 30 seconds. Flip and cook for another 30 seconds.

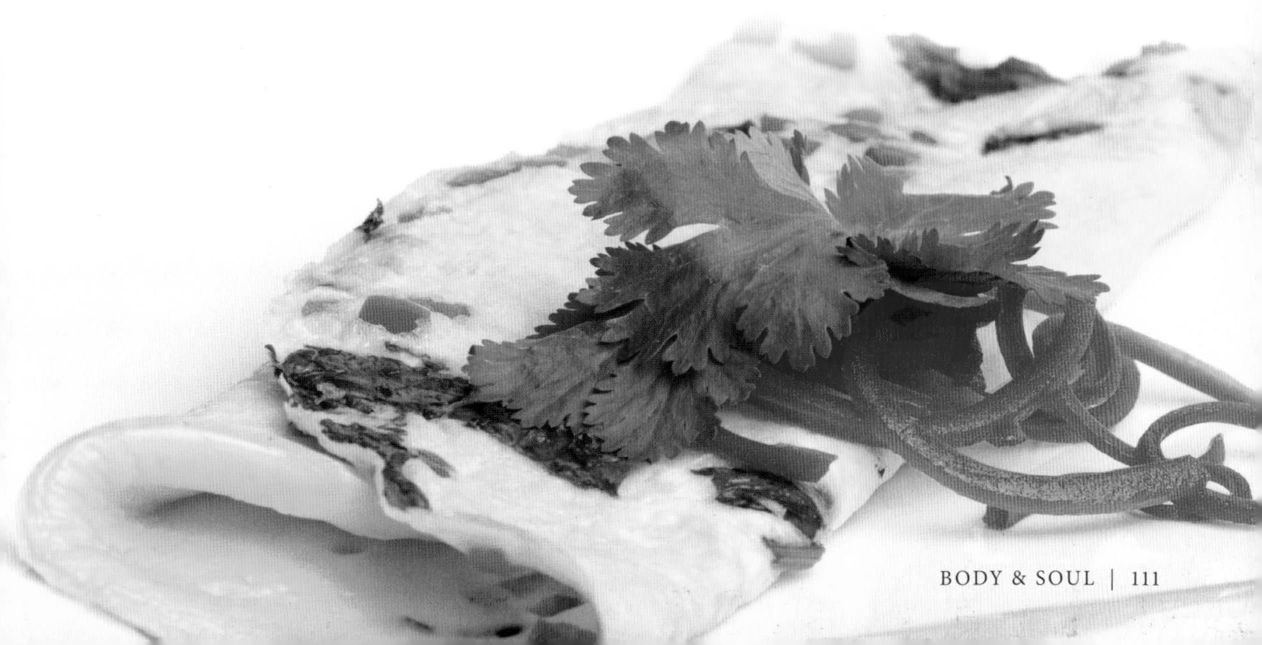

Juices & Smoothies

Not only do these liquid delights taste phenomenal, but they will boost your immune system. That means when all your buds are coming down with colds, your body will have enough internal armor to stay healthy. Sip these in the a.m. or after school.

NO-BANANA SMOOTHIE

Without the banana, this fruit 'n' veggielicious smoothie is a little less creamy. Kale is a vitamin-filled super food—and a favorite of mine at all times of the day.

SERVES 1

1 cup kale

1 large Gala apple, roughly chopped

1 English cucumber, peeled and roughly chopped

1 tbsp. fresh lemon juice

1/2 tbsp. coconut oil

4 to 5 ice cubes

Place all ingredients except ice into a high-speed blender, blend until smooth. Add ice and repeat.

MANGO-GINGER SMOOTHIE

Ginger is crazy good for digestion and is a major anti-inflammatory spice. And do I even need to mention how delicious mango is? This smoothie is yummy and powerful.

SERVES 2

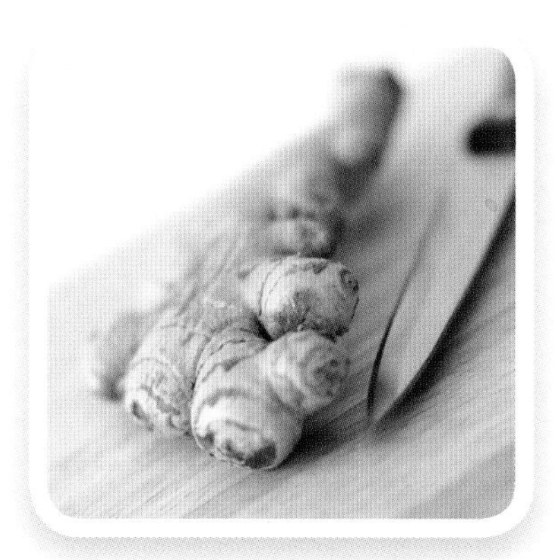

2 cups diced celery

1 diced cucumber, (about 2 cups)

1-inch chunk ginger (about the size of your thumb tip), grated

1½ cups water

2 cups parsley, loosely packed

2 cups frozen mango

1 lemon, peeled

1 tbsp. local, organic honey

Lemon to taste (use the juice of one for a real citrus boost)

Place celery, cucumber, and ginger in a juicer. Then combine the juice with all other ingredients in a blender. Mix until smooth.

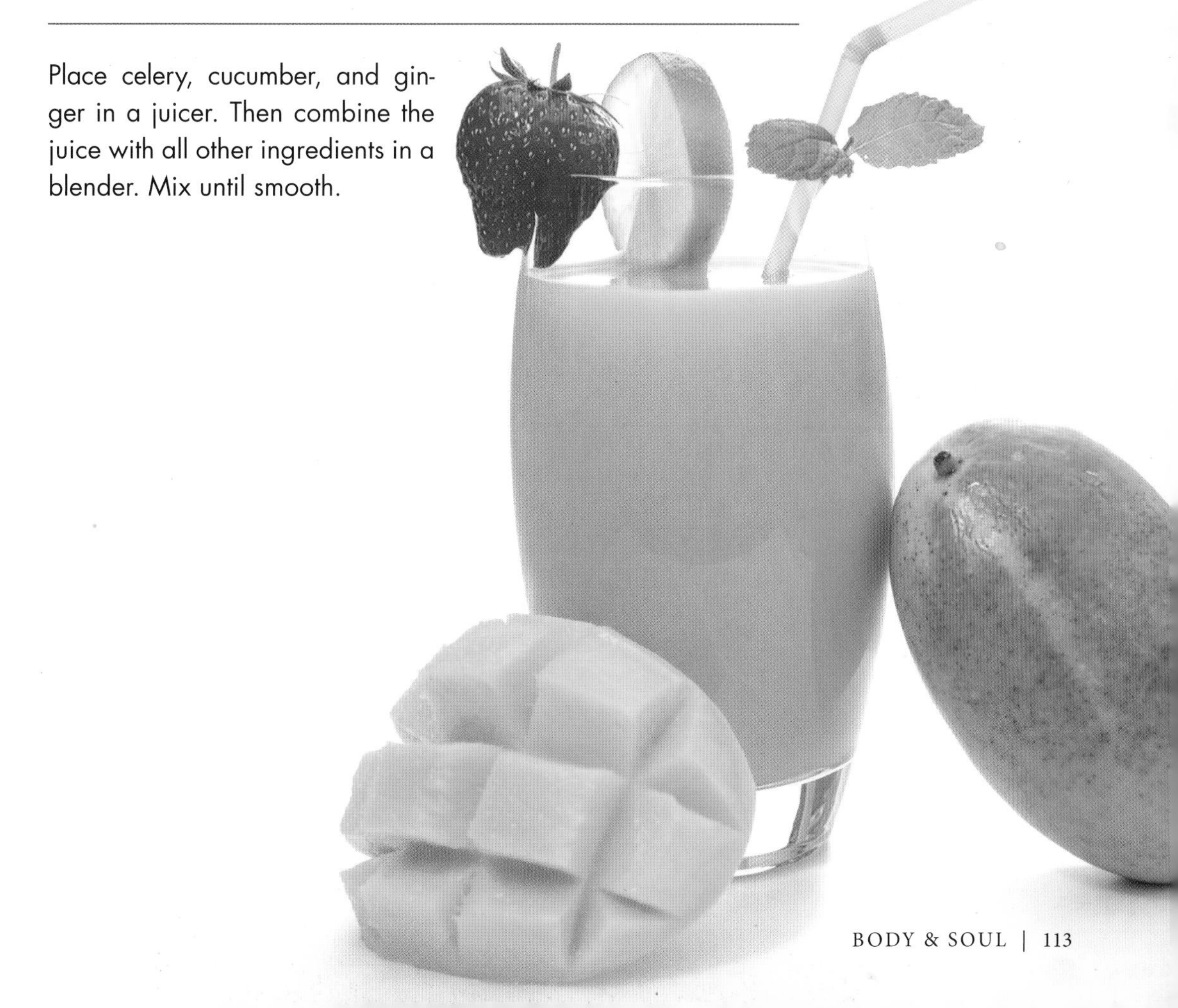

GREEN SMOOTHIE 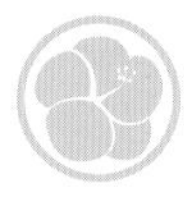

I drink a green smoothie each and every morning. Get into the habit, and it will change your life; you won't believe how much energy one drink can give you.

SERVES 1

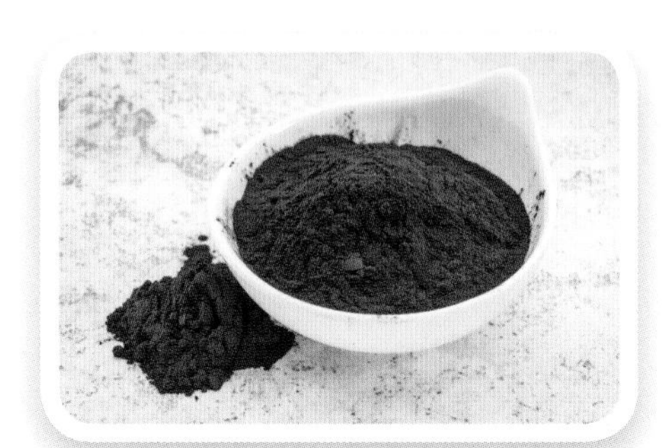

1 cup almond, rice, or coconut milk

1 cup kale

1 cup spinach

1 tsp. spirulina (powdered algae; available at health stores)

1/2 banana, frozen

1/2 pear, cored (optional — pear can be subsituted with pineapple or apple)

1 tbsp. local honey (optional)

1 tsp. ginger, grated

Place all ingredients into a blender and mix until smooth.

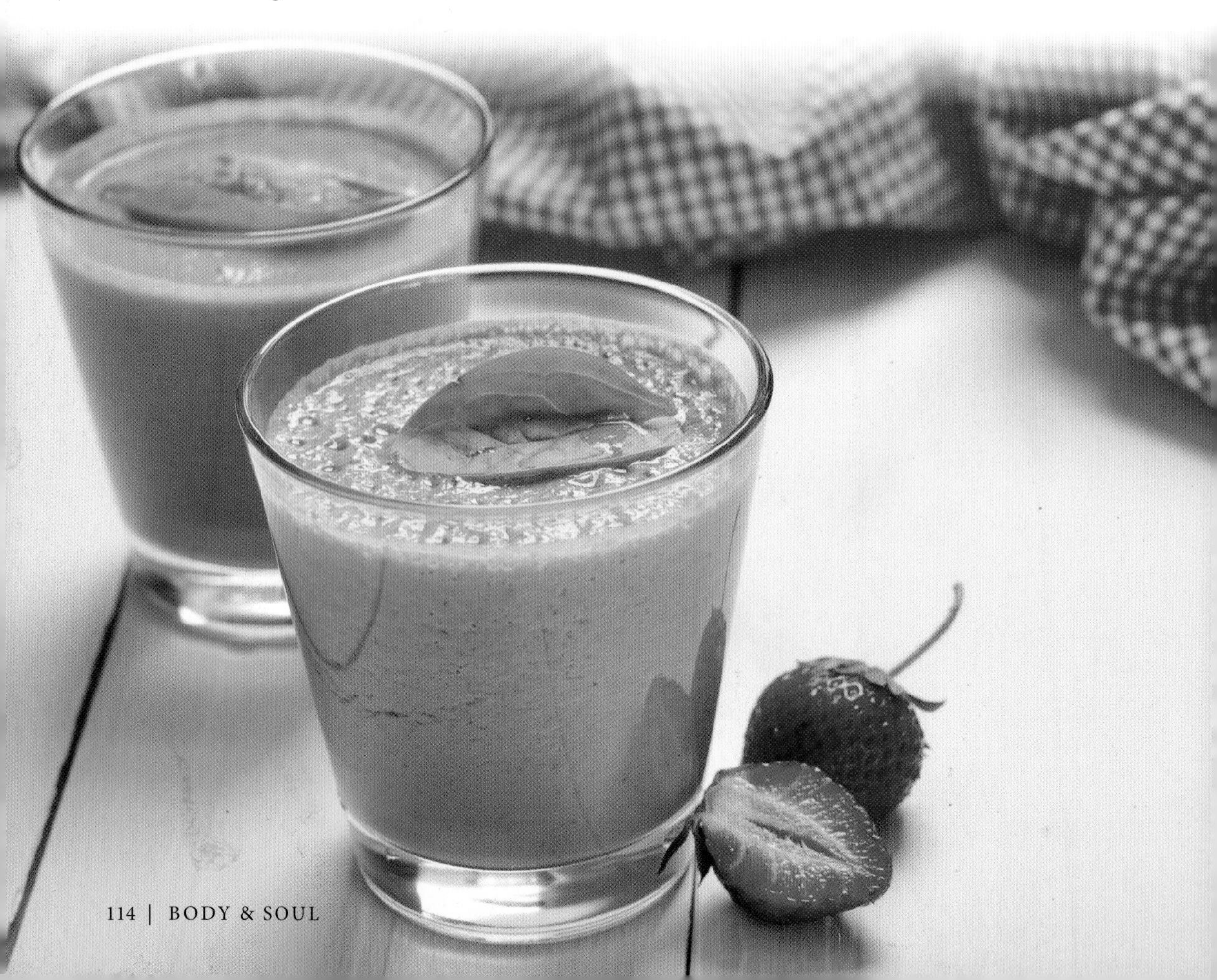

MANGO, AVOCADO, AND LIME SMOOTHIE

So rich, this smoothie is almost like a dessert.

SERVES 1

1/4 cup avocado, sliced

1 cup mango

1 tbsp. lime juice

1 tbsp. fresh mint

1 tsp. honey (optional)

2 cups crushed ice

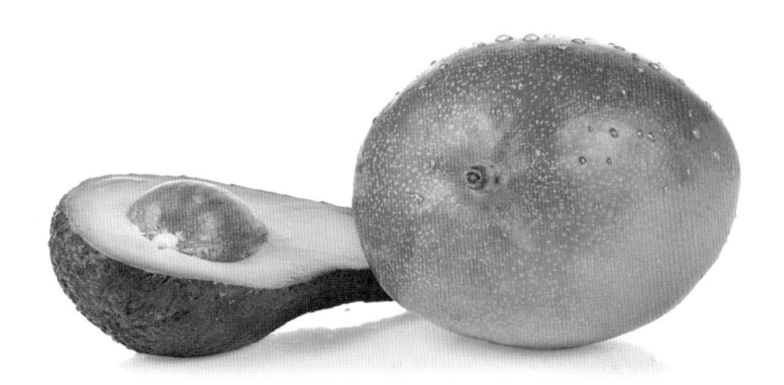

Place all ingredients into the blender (except the ice). Blend on high until smooth. Add ice and blend again.

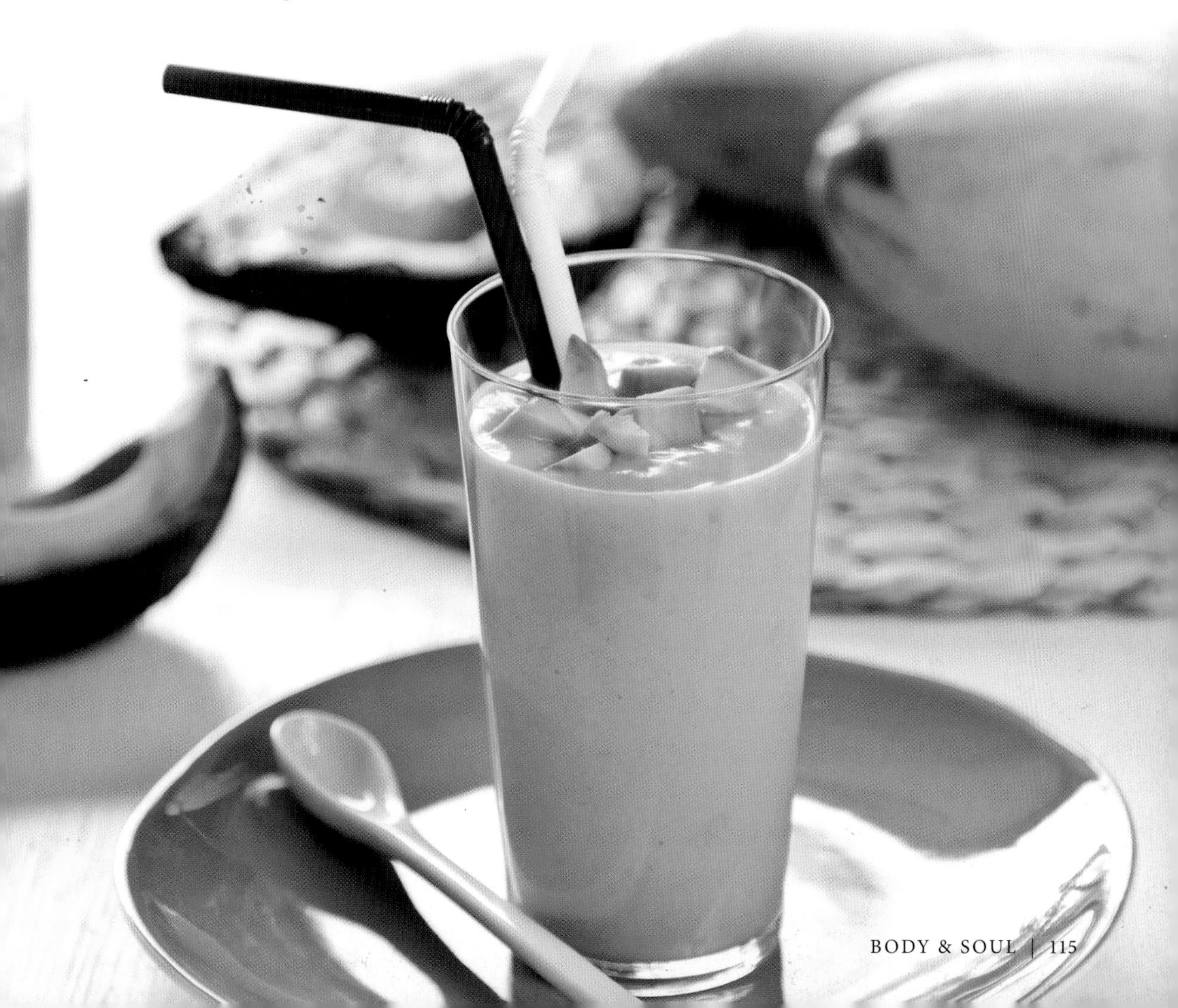

P.O.G. (PINEAPPLE ORANGE GINGER JUICE)

A twist on a Hawaiian staple, so refreshing you'll never reach for a carton of O.J. again.

SERVES 1

1 orange, peeled and juiced

1-inch chunk ginger (the size of the tip of your thumb), grated

1 cup chopped pineapple

1 splash of coconut water

Combine all ingredients in a blender and blend until smooth. Serve over ice.

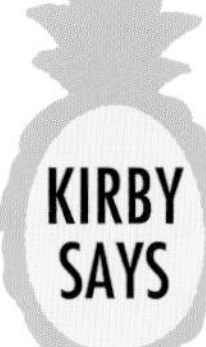

KIRBY SAYS

Ginger has a powerful taste that many of us have grown to LOVE. If this is not you, remove the ginger or reduce the amount to make it taste good for you.

BETHANY'S SOUL SECRET

Lots of people keep hand-held citrus juicers in their kitchen, so ask your parents before making this recipe. If you don't have a juicer, wash your hands really well and then roll an orange (while it's still in its peel) on the countertop. This releases some of the juice. Carefully cut the orange into four pieces and squeeze each piece over a bowl. Use a spoon to fish out the seeds.

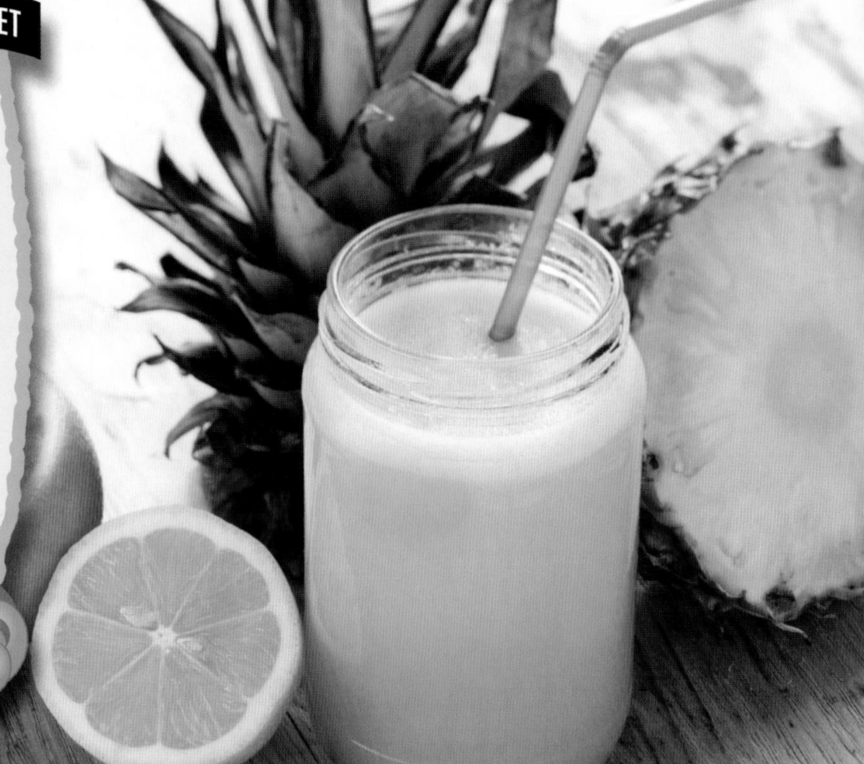

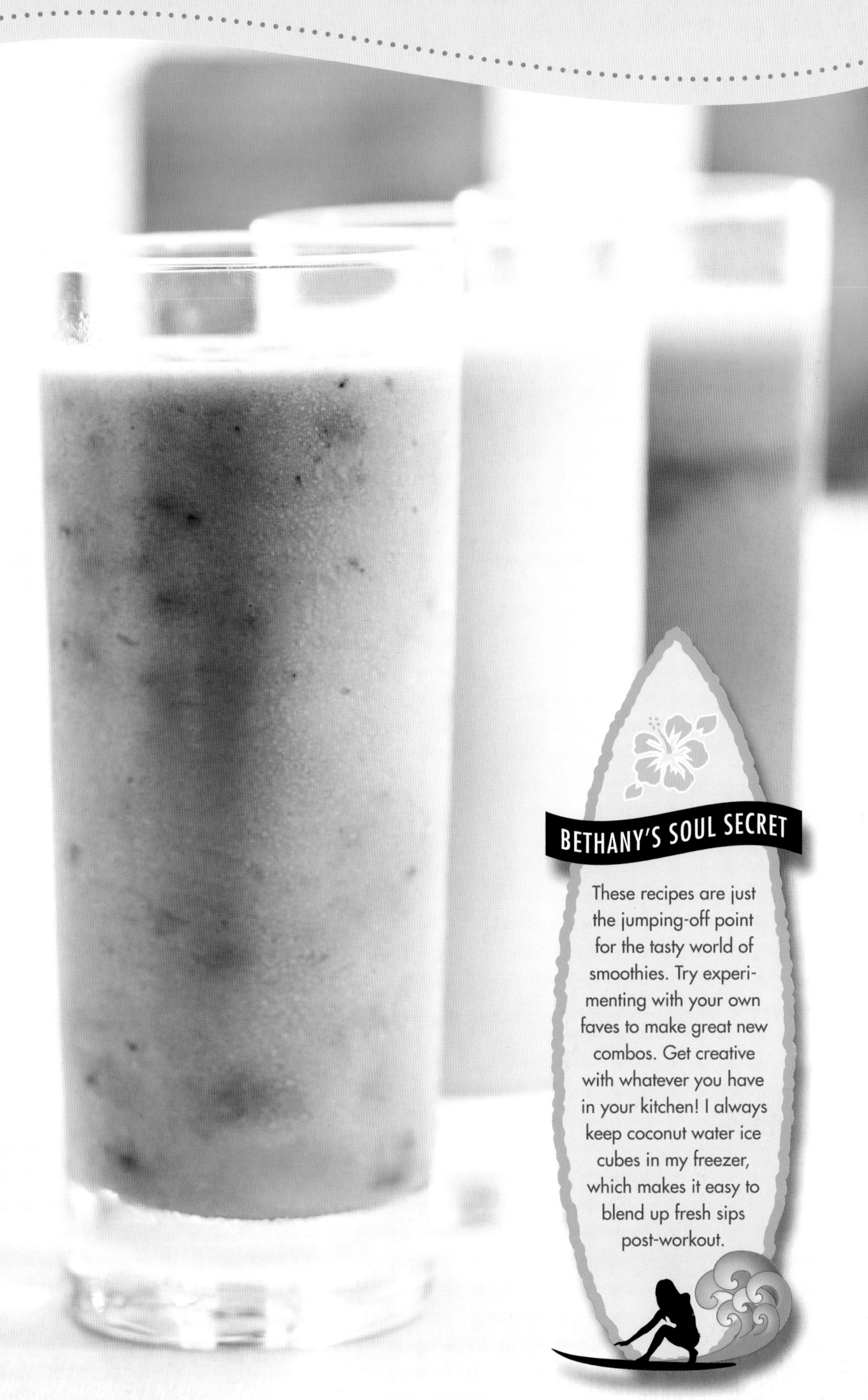

BETHANY'S SOUL SECRET

These recipes are just the jumping-off point for the tasty world of smoothies. Try experimenting with your own faves to make great new combos. Get creative with whatever you have in your kitchen! I always keep coconut water ice cubes in my freezer, which makes it easy to blend up fresh sips post-workout.

Lunch

Your midday meal is critical for re-upping your energy, but overdo it, and you can spend the rest of the day feeling bloated and tired. These recipes will restore you but leave you feeling light enough to tackle an after-school workout.

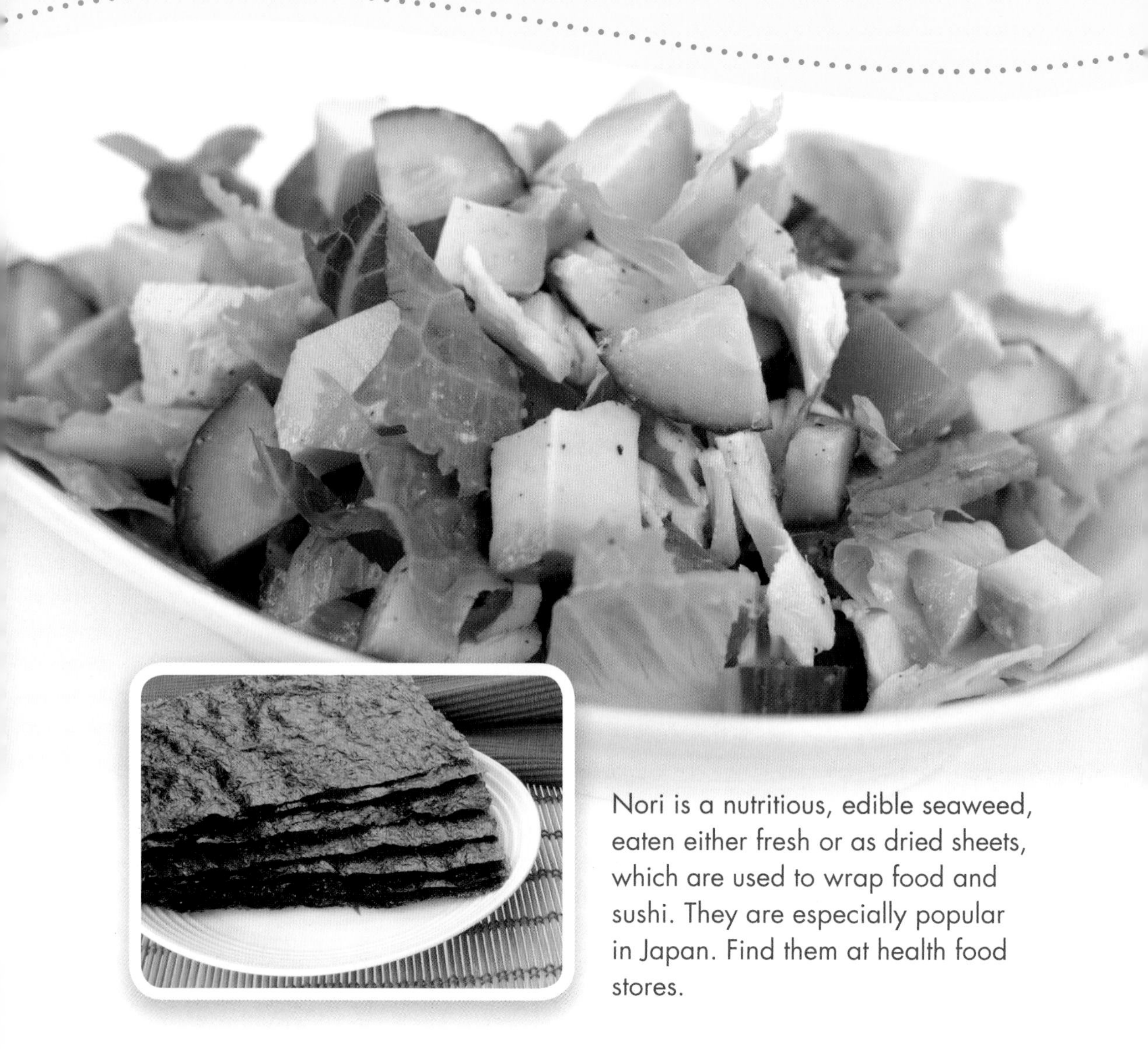

Nori is a nutritious, edible seaweed, eaten either fresh or as dried sheets, which are used to wrap food and sushi. They are especially popular in Japan. Find them at health food stores.

CHICKEN NORI WRAP

A Japanese-inspired salad with just a little bit of kick. Skip the nori if seaweed freaks you out—but I think you'll love it.

SERVES 2

FOR THE DRESSING:

Juice of 2 limes

Zest of 1 lime (just the green part of the skin, which you remove by running the lime over a fine grater)

2 tsp. coconut aminos (available at health food stores or online; also may use Braggs Liquid Aminos, available in the health food section of most grocery stores)

2 tsp. sesame oil or coconut oil

2 tsp. wasabi powder

Salt

Freshly ground pepper

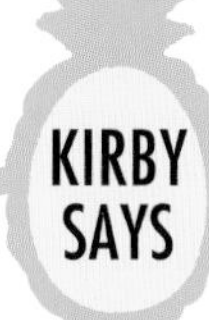

Some of my favorite coconut aminos include Braggs Liquid Aminos and Coconut Secret Raw Organic Vegan Coconut Aminos.

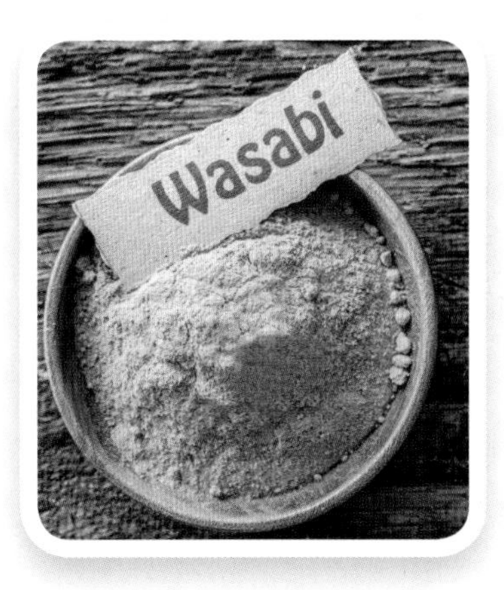

FOR THE SALAD:

1 cup cooked, organic chicken breast

1 avocado, diced

2 green onions, thinly sliced

1 tbsp. sesame seeds

Romaine or butter lettuce leaves

Nori wraps (optional)

To make the dressing, combine lime juice, lime zest, coconut aminos, sesame oil, wasabi powder, salt, and pepper in a medium bowl. Stir together and set aside.

Carefully cut the cooked chicken into chunks. Add avocado, green onion, sesame seeds, and chicken to the bowl with the dressing. Mix well. Serve atop a bed of lettuce leaves. Or wrap the mixture in lettuce leaves or nori wraps.

AHI POKE BOWL

Poke is a classic Hawaiian dish made with raw tuna. It's imperative you use sushi-grade tuna and make and eat this at home—no toting it to school! Sometimes if I'm not in the mood for raw fish, I'll sear it real quick.

SERVES 3-4

1 cup brown rice

2 large sashimi-grade ahi tuna steaks (about 1½ lbs.)

1 shallot, sliced

1/2 cup green onion, chopped

3 tbsp. Braggs Liquid Aminos or coconut aminos (available at most grocery stores; or use tamari, available in the Asian aisle of the grocery store)

1 tsp. sesame oil

1 tsp. chili garlic sauce (buy it at the grocery store)

1 tbsp. sesame seeds

1 handful greens

1 avocado, sliced

Follow instructions on package to make rice. Pat the ahi dry. Carefully cut ahi into half-inch cubes. Place in a bowl. Add shallots, green onion, Braggs sauce, sesame oil, chili garlic sauce, and sesame seeds. Gently toss. Cover and refrigerate.

Once the rice is cooked, place 1/4 of rice in a bowl, add greens of your choice (spinach, kale, etc.), add desired amount of ahi poke, and top with sliced avocado. Repeat for other servings.

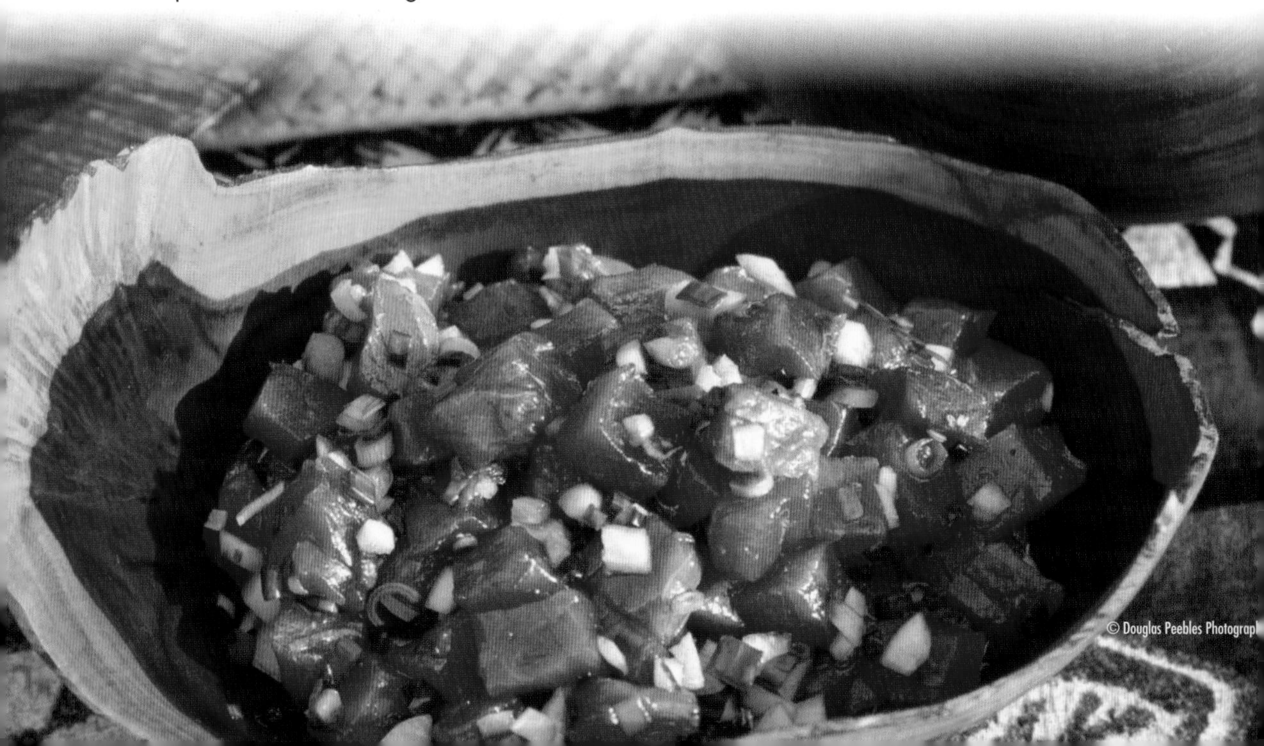

SUMMER ROLLS

It's a little hard to work with rice paper at first, but your efforts will be rewarded. These are fun to make on the weekend with your BFFs.

SERVES 4

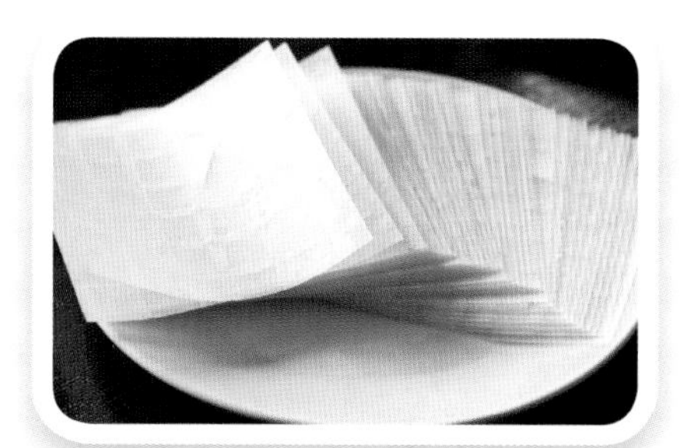

1 pack 6½ inch rice paper round (found near Asian foods)

1 bowl of very hot water

1 yellow bell pepper, cut into squares, ribs and seeds removed

1 head green leaf lettuce, leaves separated

1 avocado, sliced lengthwise into strips

1 cucumber, thinly sliced

2 carrots, thinly sliced

2 to 3 leaves red cabbage, shredded (optional)

Prepare rice paper by dipping one round at a time into very hot water until soft (about 5 seconds). Remove rice paper from the water and spread it flat on a clean work surface. Lay the yellow bell pepper over the bottom third of the rice paper, flattening it with your palm. Add green leaf lettuce and top with avocado, cucumber, carrots, and red cabbage.

Fold in the left and the right sides of the rice paper; lift the bottom edge over the vegetables. Tightly tuck and roll the rice paper away from you. Continue rolling as tightly as possible until the roll is closed. Set aside, seam side down, on a plate, then cover with a damp towel (to prevent drying).

Repeat until you've used all the vegetables. You can refrigerate the rolls, covered with the damp towel until ready to be served. They can be kept in the fridge for 2 to 3 hours before serving. To serve, cut each roll crosswise into desired size and serve with tamari sauce.

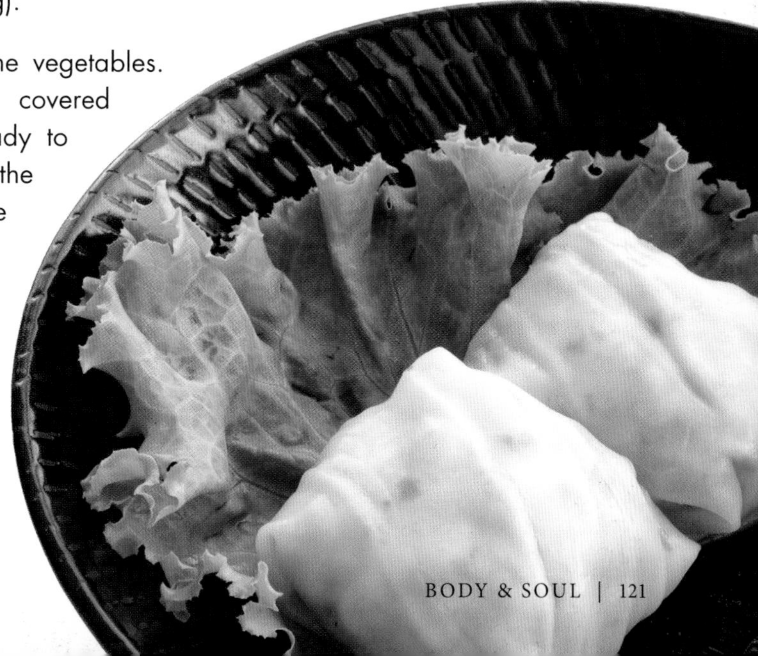

Theme Salads

Many people ask me how I can eat salads every day and not "get sick of it." My answer revolves around making my daily salad around a "theme." If I am in the mood for Mexican, I make a Mexican salad. If I am in the mood for Greek food, I make a Greek salad–can you see where I'm going? Here are some ideas for theme salads that are easy to put together, and they taste great. First start with some local organic greens. Then add the interesting ingredients found here.

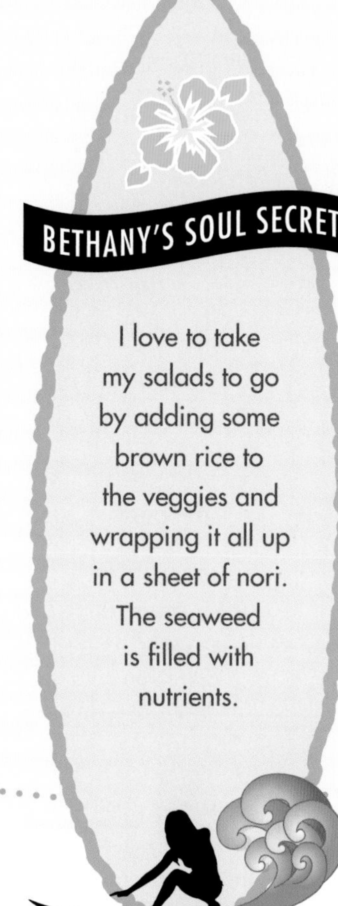

MEXICAN SALAD

Black beans, organic corn kernels, chopped green onion, a little grated natural cheese, avocado, diced onion, tomatoes, salt and pepper to taste. Add a natural salsa and squeeze some lime juice over salad as a dressing.

GREEK SALAD

Cherry or Roma tomatoes, diced onion, chopped cucumber, olives, and crumbled feta cheese. Toss with a vinaigrette dressing.

ITALIAN SALAD

Chopped Italian olives, julienne-sliced sun-dried tomatoes, and shredded mozzarella cheese. Toss with a vinaigrette or natural Italian dressing.

Homemade Salad Dressings

There are a million different salad dressings to buy in the store, but many are filled with partially-hydrogenated oils and lots of other preservatives. Besides, making your own is crazy easy.

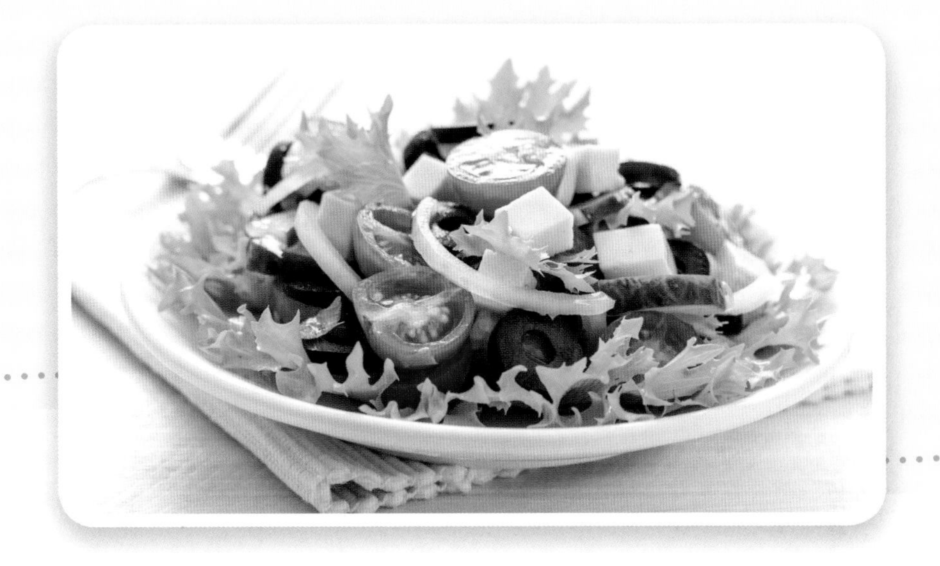

BASIC DRESSING

3 tbsp. fresh-squeezed lemon juice

1 ½ cups coconut oil or olive oil

1 clove garlic, crushed

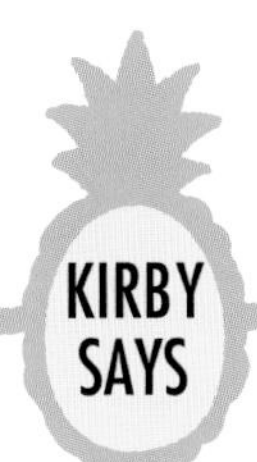

KIRBY SAYS

Using a blender will result in a much creamier dressing. Keep covered in the fridge for up to a week.

CAESAR SALAD DRESSING

1/2 cup virgin olive oil

1/2 cup coconut oil

1 tbsp. fresh lemon juice

2 tbsp. red wine vinegar

2 to 3 fresh garlic cloves, minced

1 tsp. prepared mustard

1 tsp. tamari sauce

2 tbsp. Parmesan cheese (or ground sunflower seeds if you want a dairy-free dressing)

Pick a dressing. Place all ingredients into a blender and mix well, or place in a bowl and whisk with a fork.

Dinner

Between school and extracurriculars, cooking in the evening can feel like a chore. Instead, use the time spent chopping and sautéing to give your mind a break and commune with God. We can reflect how blessed we are to have food to eat, how God in his infinite wisdom has created plants that produce such wonderful flavors. We can also use this time to ask God to bless us with good health as we prepare and consume the food.

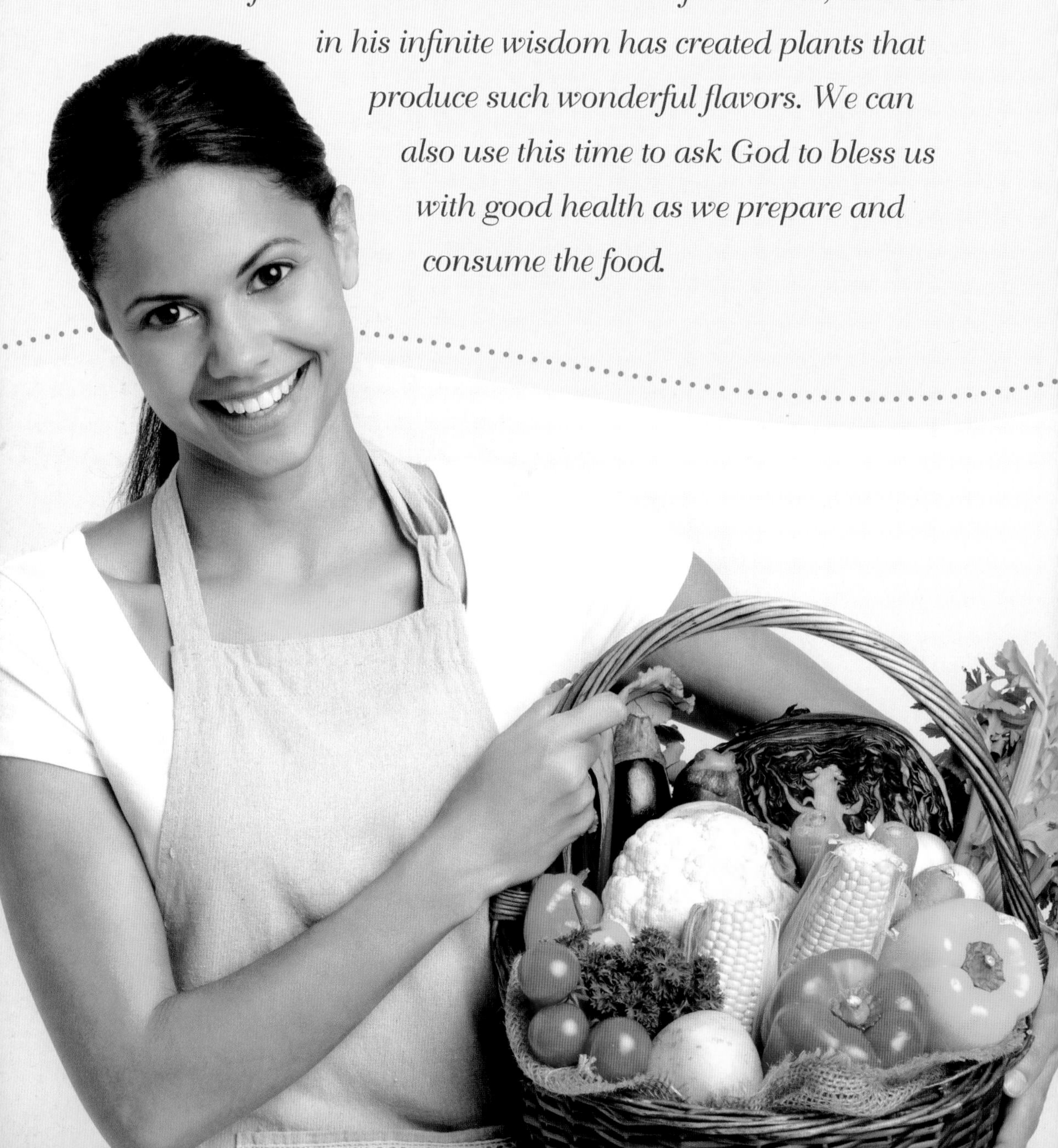

MACADAMIA NUT CRUSTED CHICKEN

Macadamia nuts are super popular in Hawaii and an excellent source of good fat. Trust me, you'll love this one.

SERVES 4

1/2 cup chopped macadamia nuts

4 to 6 ounce portions of organic chicken breast per serving

Fine sea salt

1 large organic egg white

2 tbsp. coconut oil or olive oil

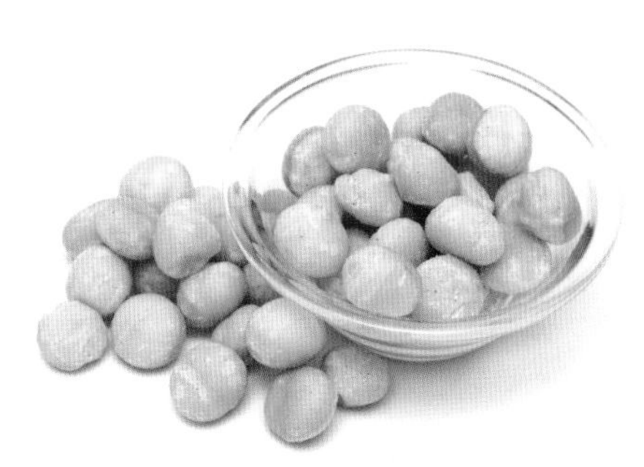

Preheat oven to 375°F. Lightly coat baking dish with coconut oil. Grind macadamia nuts in a food processor on "chop" speed—be careful not to grind them to a paste. Transfer nuts to a wide, shallow bowl. Season both sides of chicken with a little sea salt.

Whisk egg white in another wide, shallow bowl until frothy. Dip top of each fillet in egg white, then into macadamia nuts, pressing to adhere. Place chicken into prepared baking dish. Bake for 20 to 30 minutes or until chicken is white all the way through. The macadamia nuts should be toasted and brown. If they're not, turn oven to broil for 1 minute at the end so the nuts get golden brown.

Serve on a bed of organic mixed greens with a side of grilled veggies.

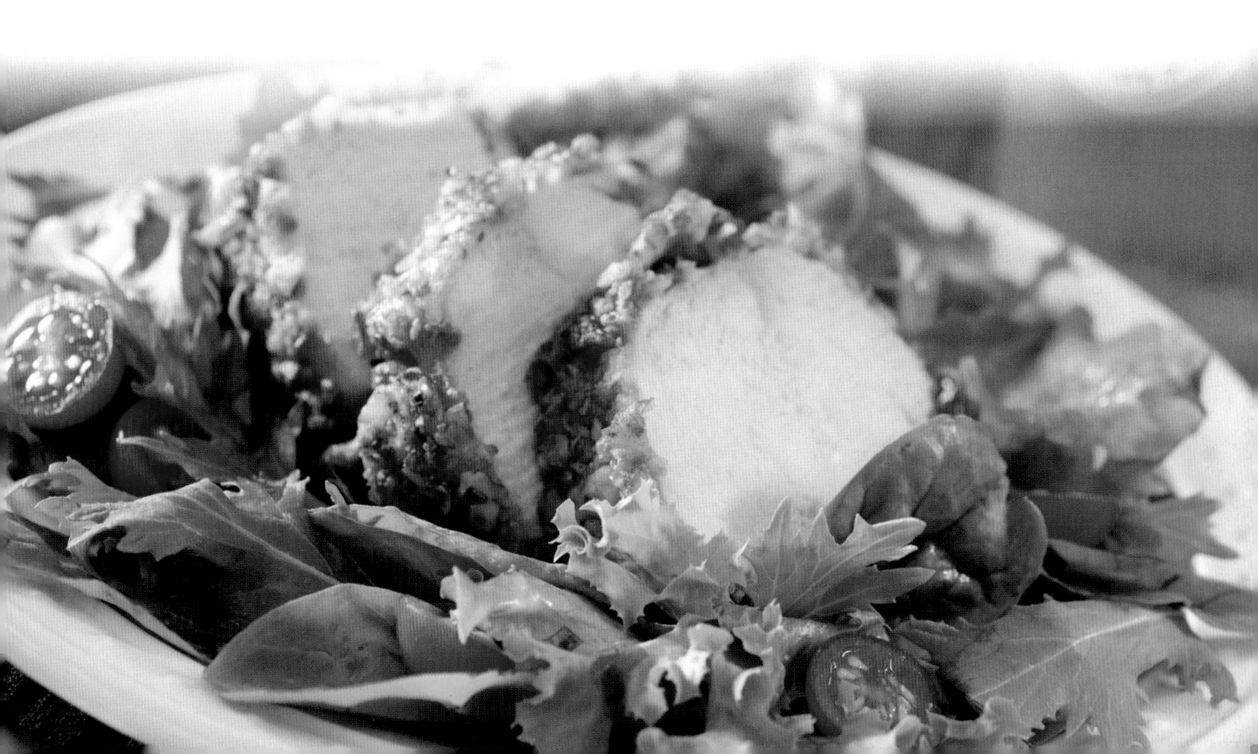

GRILLED FISH WITH MANGO-AVOCADO SALSA

Just a little sweet, this fish works on a salad or stuffed into a lettuce wrap.

SERVES 4

1 medium ripe mango, peeled and diced into 1/2-inch cubes

1 medium ripe avocado, peeled and diced into 1/2-inch cubes

1 cup cherry tomatoes, quartered

Fresh cilantro, thinly sliced to taste

3 tbsp. coconut oil, divided (1 tbsp. for salsa, 2 tbsp. for fish)

3 tbsp. fresh lime juice, divided

1/4–1/2 cup unsweetened coconut shavings

Sea salt

Freshly ground black pepper

4 6-ounce fish (mahi-mahi, halibut, ahi, cod)

Heat grill to medium-high (if using a grill pan on the stove, wait to heat it).

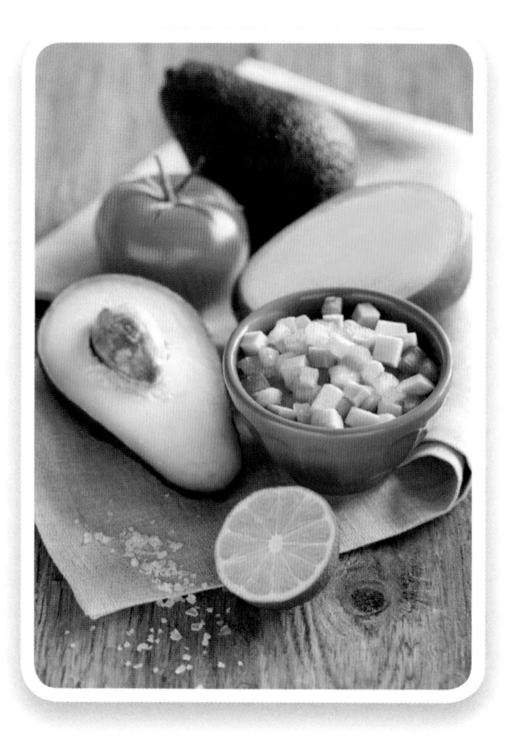

Combine salsa ingredients in a large bowl: mango, avocado, tomatoes, cilantro, 1 tablespoon oil, and 1 tablespoon lime juice. Season salsa to taste with coconut shavings, salt, and pepper. Set aside at room temperature; toss gently occasionally.

Place fish fillets in a glass baking dish. Drizzle about 2 tablespoons of oil and 2 tablespoons of lime juice over fish and season with salt and pepper. Let marinate at room temperature for about 10 minutes, turning fish occasionally.

Make sure grill rack is brushed with oil before placing fish on it. Grill fish just until opaque in center, about 5 minutes per side.

Spoon fresh, homemade salsa over fish; add more lime juice and coconut shavings if desired. Serve on a bed of organic mixed greens or in a lettuce wrap.

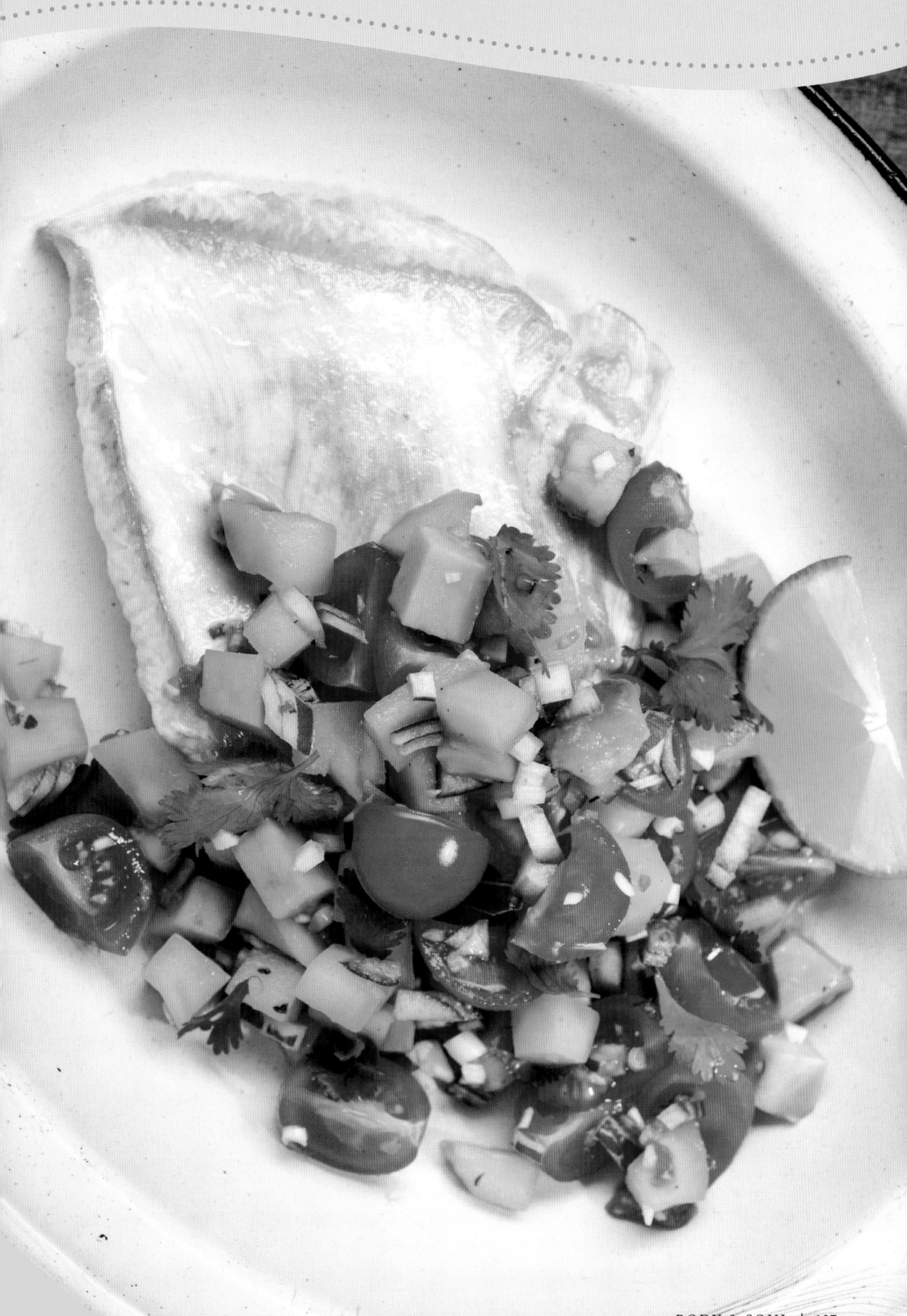

TACO SALAD

Traditional taco spice packets are packed with sodium. This recipe has plenty of flavor but is a zillion times better for you.

SERVES 4

BEEF MIXTURE

1 1/3 lbs. organic ground beef

1 tsp. coconut oil

1 tsp. chili powder (or to taste)

3 garlic cloves, minced

1/2 white onion, chopped

1/2 tsp. salt

Freshly ground black pepper to taste

FOR THE SALAD

1 head green leaf lettuce (organic) or other lettuce, thinly sliced

1 red bell pepper, chopped

1/2 white onion, chopped

1 cup cherry tomatoes, quartered

1 can organic, unsalted baby corn, drained

1 can organic black beans, rinsed

1 avocado, cut into 1/2-inch cubes

1 bunch cilantro, chopped

Juice of 1 lime

Sea salt and freshly ground black pepper to taste

To make beef mixture, warm pan over medium-high heat, add oil, chili powder, and minced garlic and stir. Add onion and coat onion with oil. Add beef to the center of the pan—use a stiff spatula to break the ground meat into several pieces. Continue crumbling meat into smaller pieces. Add salt and pepper. Stir occasionally until beef is no longer pink.

In a large bowl, mix the salad ingredients, toss, and set aside. Add desired amount of ground beef on top of your salad. Add more lime juice for dressing or use homemade guacamole (page 132).

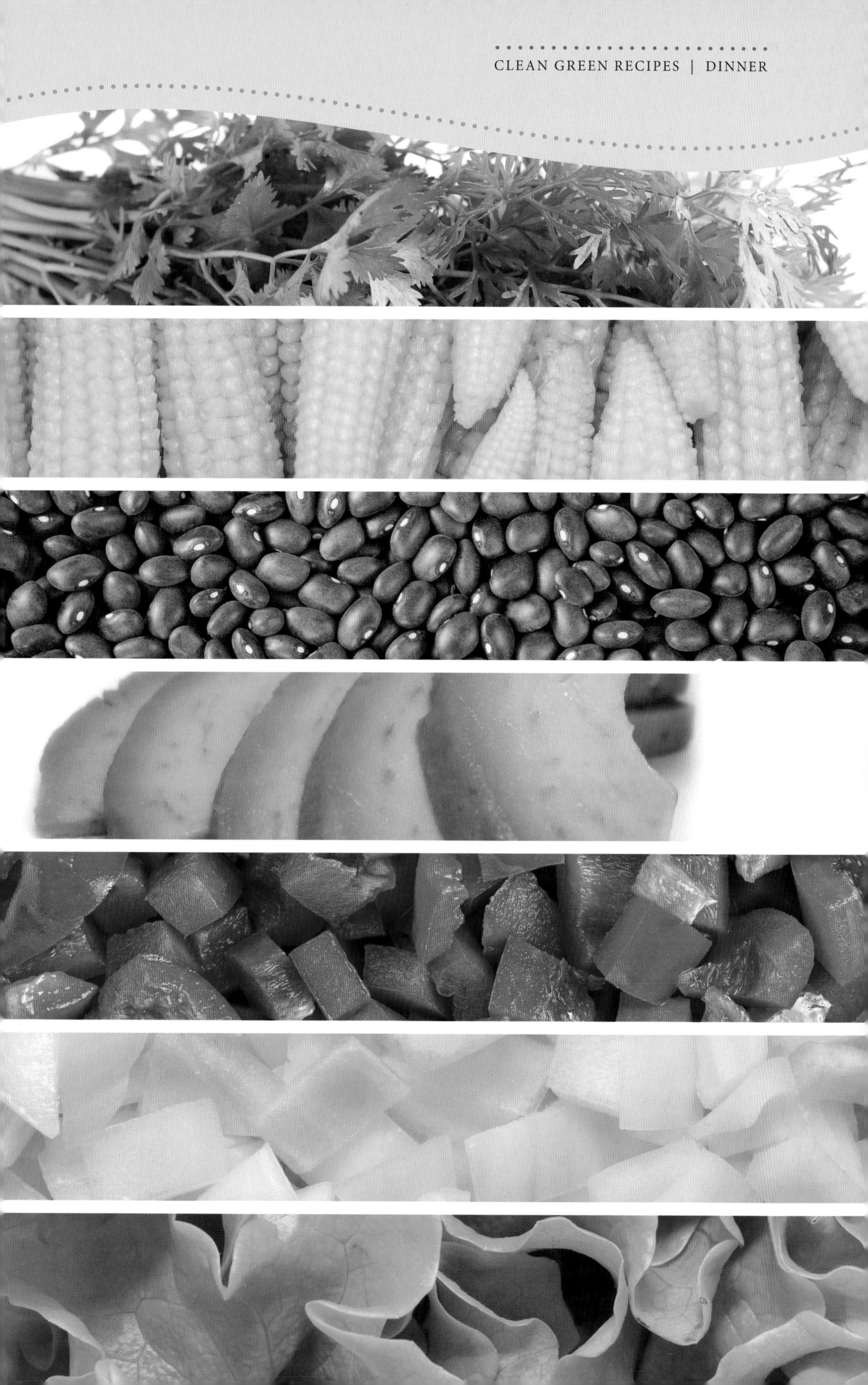

GRILLED VEGGIE SALAD

A no-brainer for vegetarians or for those times when you just need a giant salad (after a big lunch, perhaps?).

SERVES 4 TO 6

FOR THE SALAD

- 2 medium zucchini, halved lengthwise, ends removed
- 2 medium yellow squash, halved lengthwise, ends removed
- 1 pound asparagus spears
- 2 tbsp. coconut oil
- 1 pint cherry tomatoes, halved
- 1 head lettuce, shredded
- 1/4 cup chopped fresh basil

FOR THE DRESSING

- 1/4 cup chopped fresh basil leaves
- 2 tbsp. fresh lemon juice
- 1 tbsp. Dijon mustard
- 1 tsp. honey
- 1/4 tsp. salt
- 1/4 cup coconut oil or olive oil

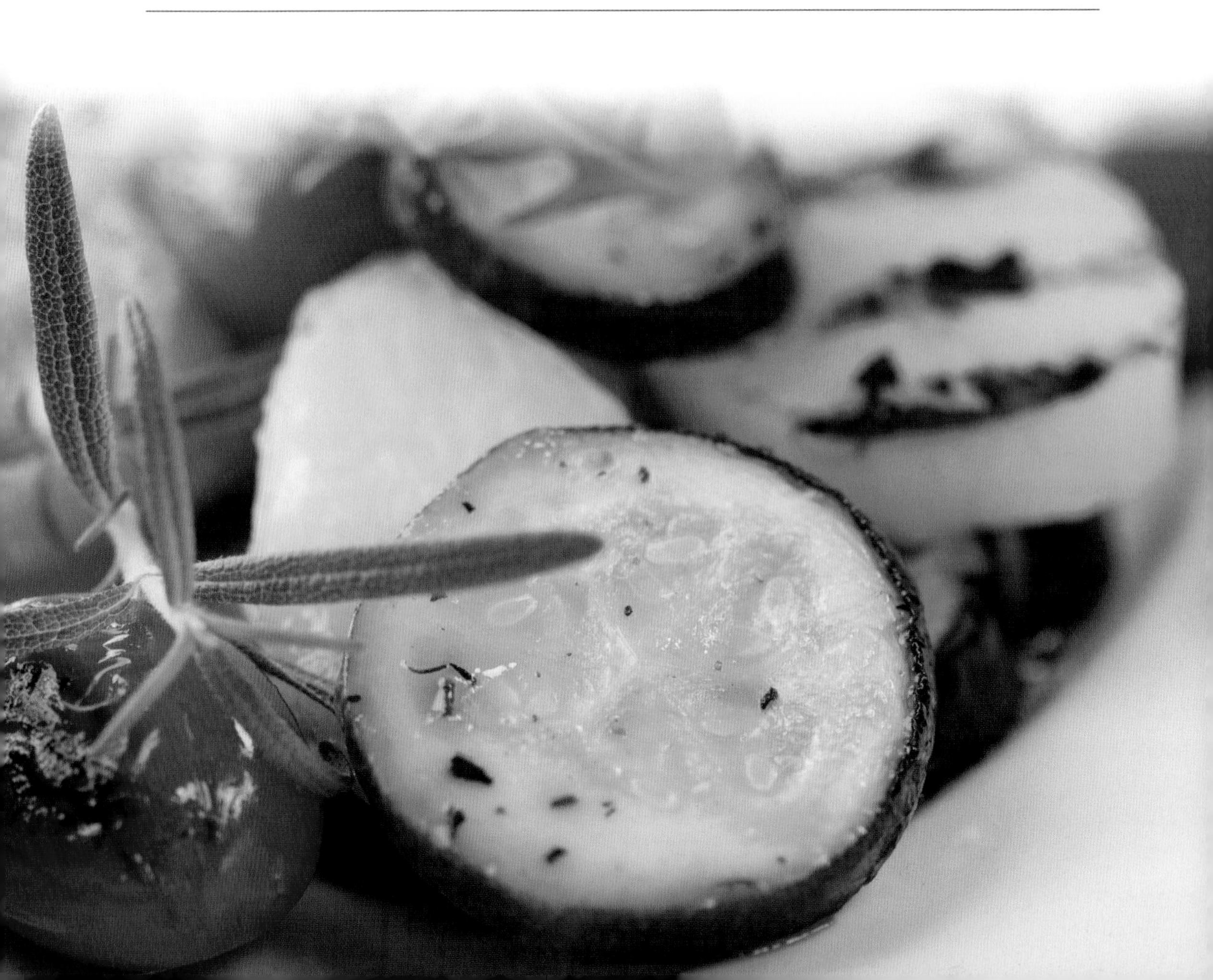

Preheat grill. Brush zucchini, squash, and asparagus lightly with coconut oil, and sprinkle lightly with salt and pepper. Put veggies on the hot grill and cook until tender and lightly charred (flip halfway through). Depending on the thickness, it can take between 10 and 20 minutes.

Remove cooked veggies from grill with tongs (be careful!) and let cool to room temperature. Cut squash and zucchini in large chunks and place in large bowl. Cut asparagus spears into one-inch pieces and discard ends. Add to bowl. Add halved cherry tomatoes, shredded lettuce, and chopped basil into the large bowl. Toss salad until well mixed.

In a blender or food processor, combine all dressing ingredients except oil. Cover blender and pulse a few times until ingredients are combined. Turn blender on low, open pour spout, and slowly add oil. Mixture will splash as it thickens, so be careful. Turn off the blender and scrape sides. Give it one last whirl.

Add dressing to the salad, and toss until veggies are well coated. Add a source of protein (chicken, fish, steak) if desired.

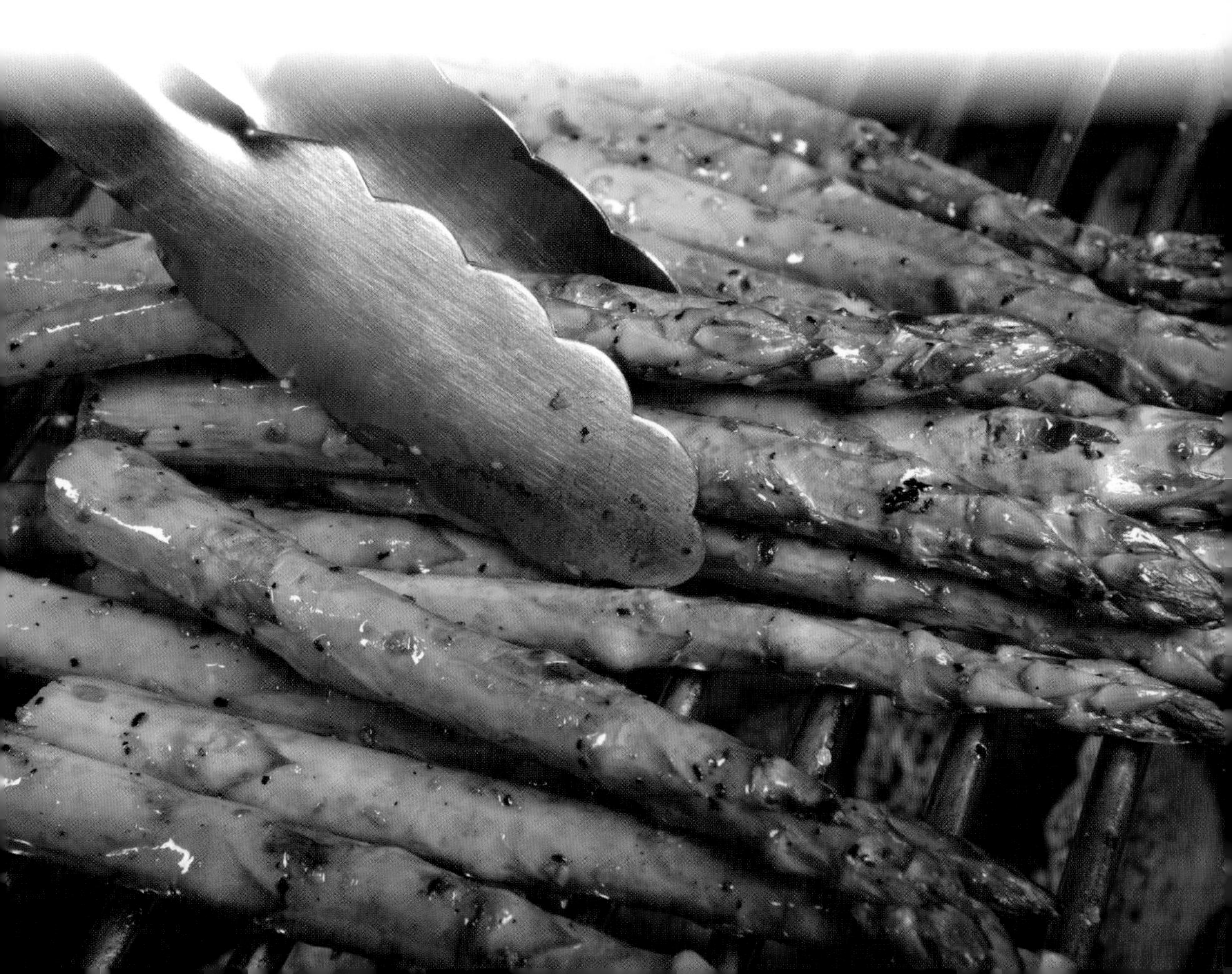

Side Dishes

Sometimes when girls start eating healthy, they actually don't eat enough. They get hungry and reach for junk later. Stave off late-night munching by boosting your entrée with a side of something amazing.

HOMEMADE GUACAMOLE

A crowd-pleaser with taco salad or, well, anything.

SERVES 4

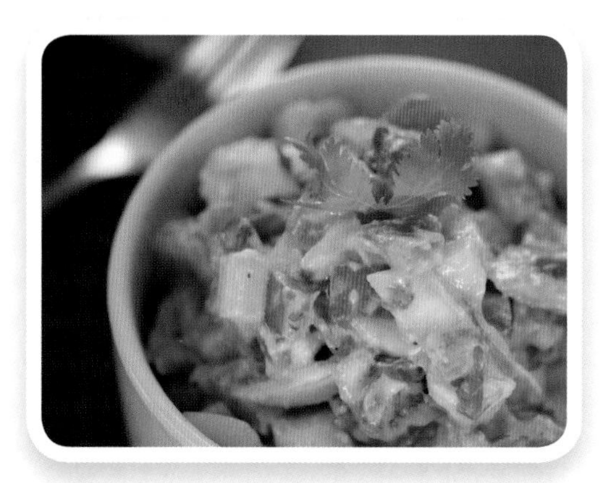

1 medium ripe avocado, peeled and cut into 1/2-inch cubes

Juice from 1 lime

1 garlic clove, minced (optional)

1/4 white onion, chopped

1/4 cup cherry tomatoes, quartered

Small bunch of fresh cilantro, finely chopped

1/4 teaspoon salt (or to taste)

1/4 teaspoon fresh ground pepper (or to taste)

Split avocado and remove pit; use a spoon to scoop avocado flesh and place in a mixing bowl. With a fork, smash the avocado. Add lime juice and continue to smash the avocado until creamy (adding more or less lime). Add garlic, onion, cilantro, and tomato. Season with salt, pepper, and more lime if desired.

OVEN-ROASTED BROCCOLI (OR ANY VEGGIES, REALLY)

Even broccoli haters will fall for this tempting plate of greens.

SERVES 2 TO 4 AS A SIDE DISH

1 bunch broccoli

3 to 5 garlic cloves, minced

2 tbsp. coconut oil or olive oil

1/2 tsp. sea salt

Heat oven to 400°F. Wash and cut broccoli—keep stems. In a large bowl, toss broccoli, oil, minced garlic, and salt. Spread broccoli on a parchment-lined baking sheet. Bake 12 to15 minutes until slightly browned and tender.

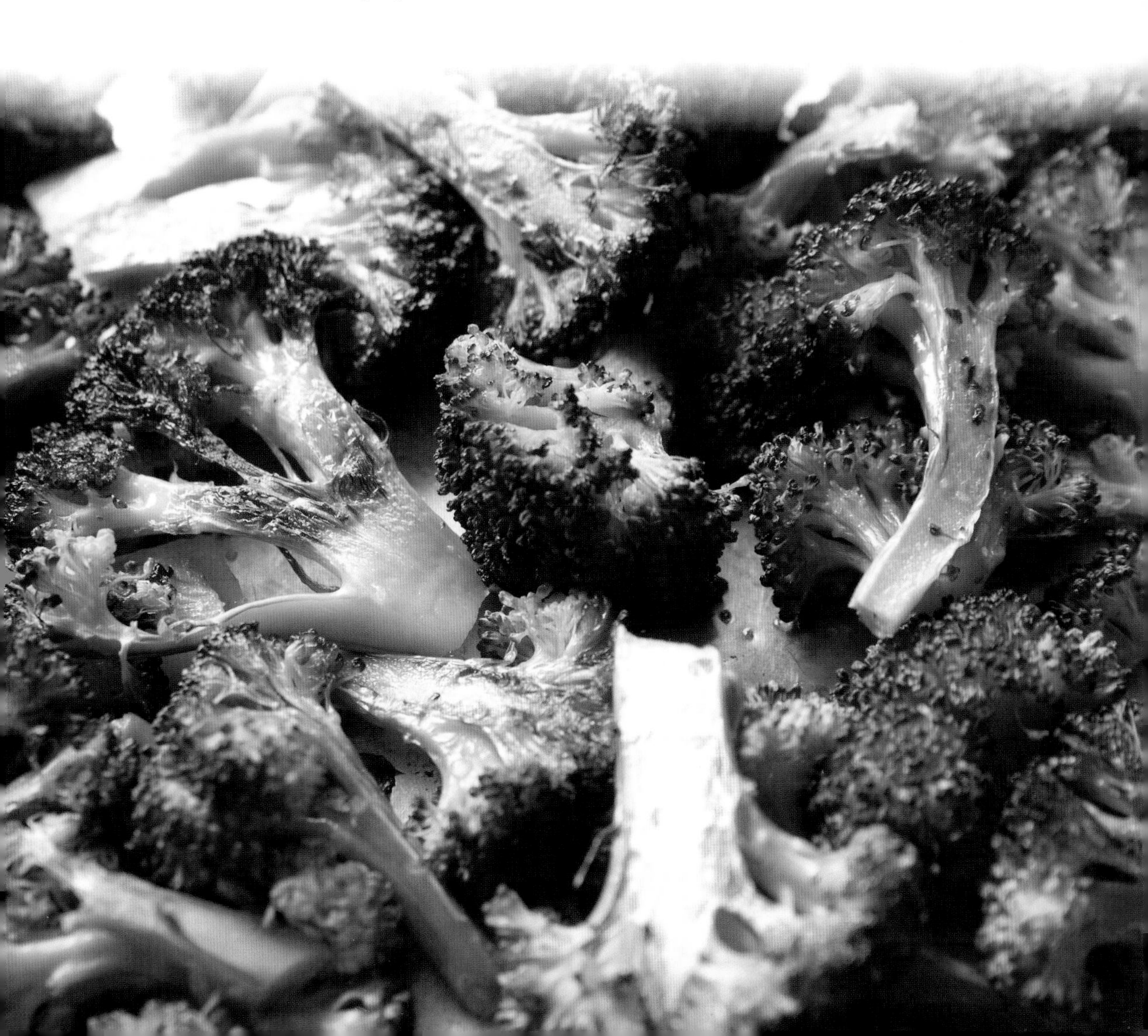

OVEN-ROASTED ASPARAGUS

These spears have a surprising bit of sweetness (just a little) and are great with macadamia-crusted chicken.

SERVES 4 AS A SIDE DISH

1 bunch asparagus

2 tbsp. coconut oil or olive oil

1/4 tsp. sea salt

Heat oven to 350°F. Wash asparagus and trim dried parts from the bottom. Pat dry. Line up asparagus side by side, in a single layer on a parchment-lined baking dish. Drizzle oil, roll asparagus, and then sprinkle with salt. Bake for 10 to 12 minutes until the tips start to turn brown.

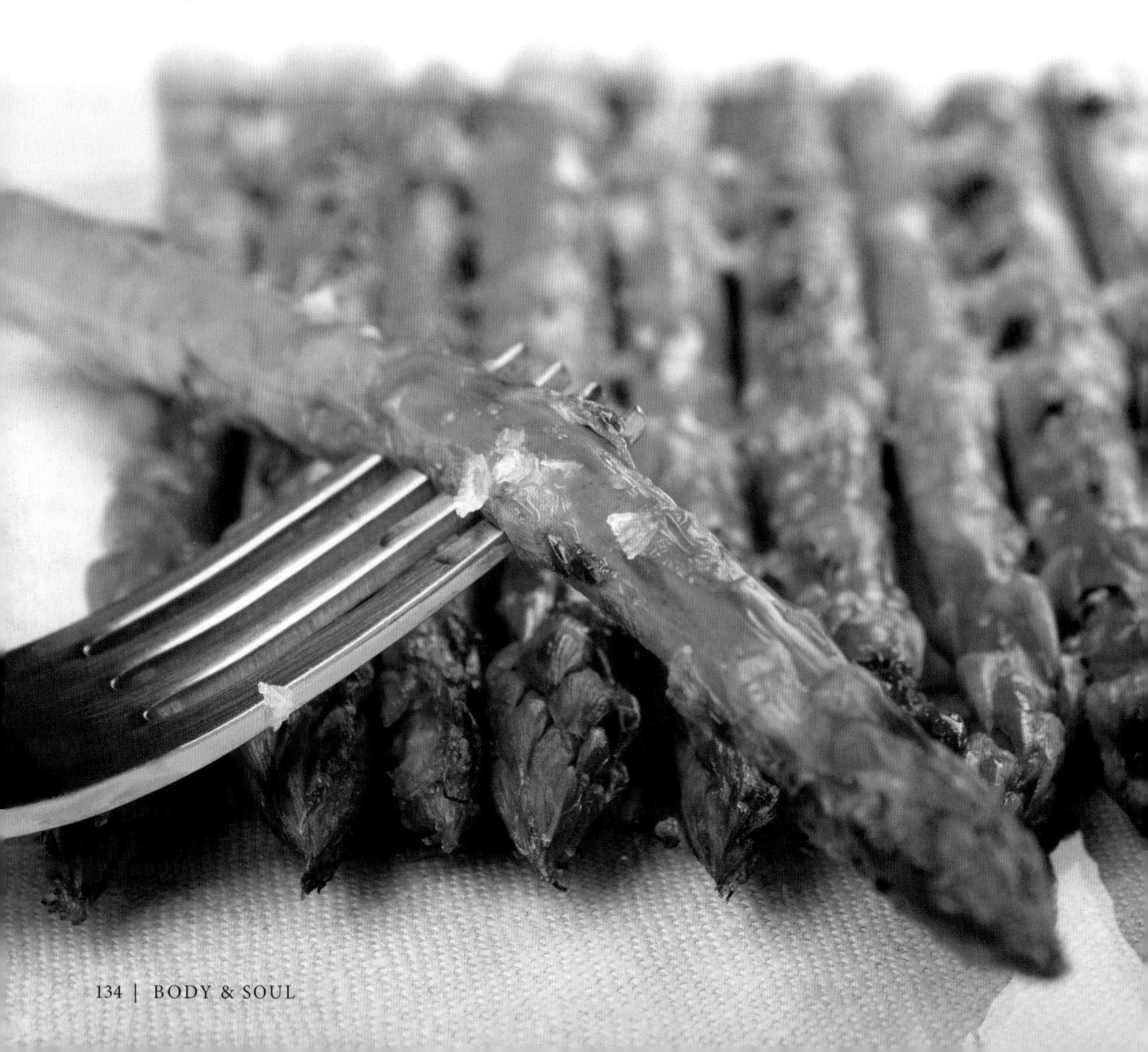

VEGGIE QUINOA OR BROWN RICE

With a salad, you could have this dish for lunch any day of the week.

SERVES 2 AS A SIDE DISH

1 cup quinoa (or brown rice)

2 tbsp. coconut oil

4 garlic cloves, minced

1/2 white onion, chopped

1/2 red bell pepper, chopped

1/2 tsp. sea salt

1/2 tsp. freshly ground black pepper

Cook quinoa in a small pot or rice cooker (follow instructions on package). Heat coconut oil over medium heat in a large skillet. Add garlic, onion, and bell pepper. Sauté until soft. Once quinoa is cooked, stir in bell pepper, onion, and garlic mixture. Season with salt and pepper.

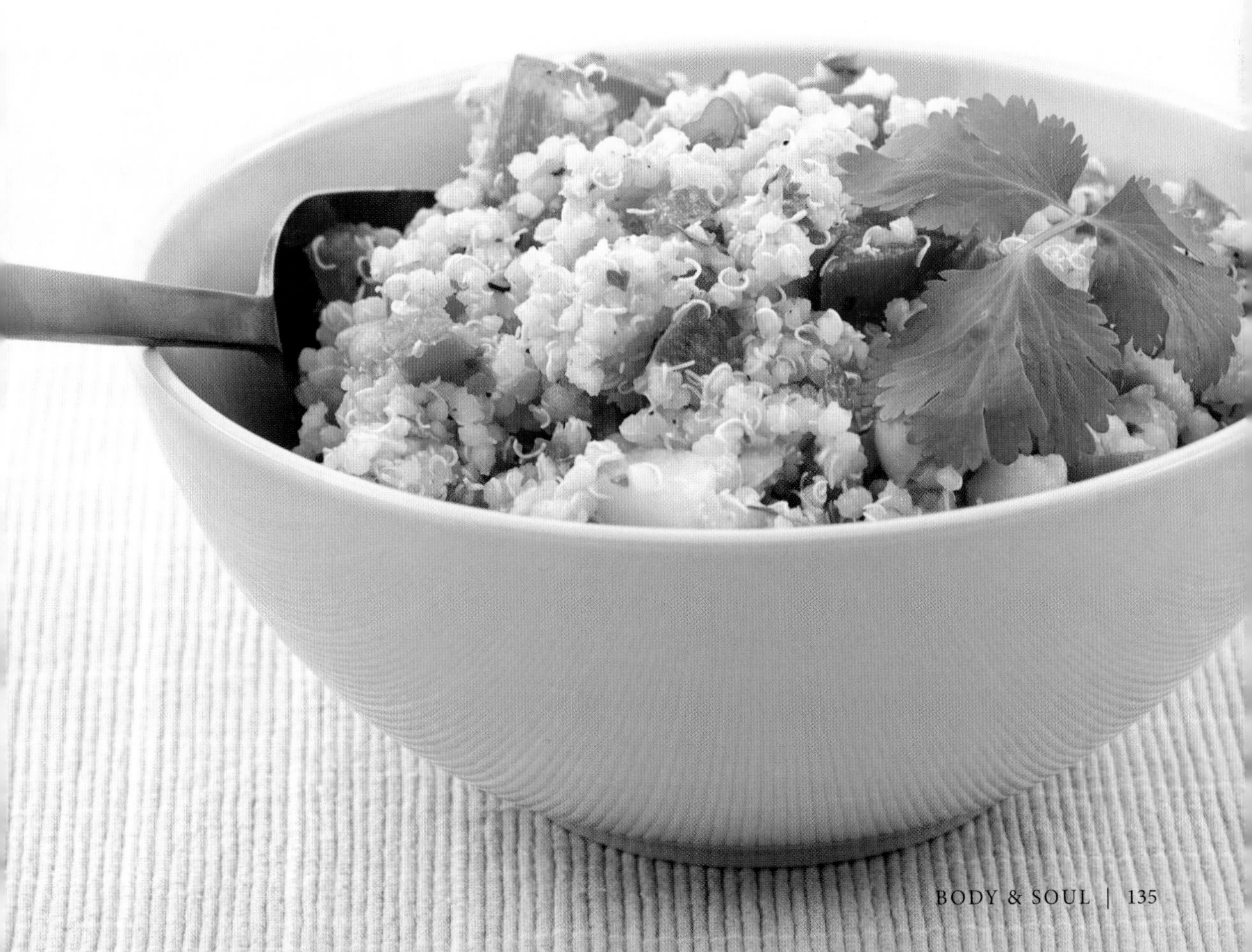

PURPLE SWEET POTATOES

The purple ones are a real treat, but you can use regular sweet potatoes (or yams) too.

SERVES 2 TO 4 AS A SIDE DISH

2 to 3 large purple sweet potatoes, peeled and chopped

1 cup coconut cream or milk

Salt to taste

1/4 tsp. ground cinnamon (optional)

Grated fresh ginger to taste (optional)

Coconut shavings to taste (optional)

Place potatoes in a large pot. Fill with water and cover on high heat. Boil for 25 to 30 minutes. Drain potatoes and place them back into the pot. Add coconut cream and a pinch of salt, then mash with a potato masher until desired consistency. Stir in the extras and serve.

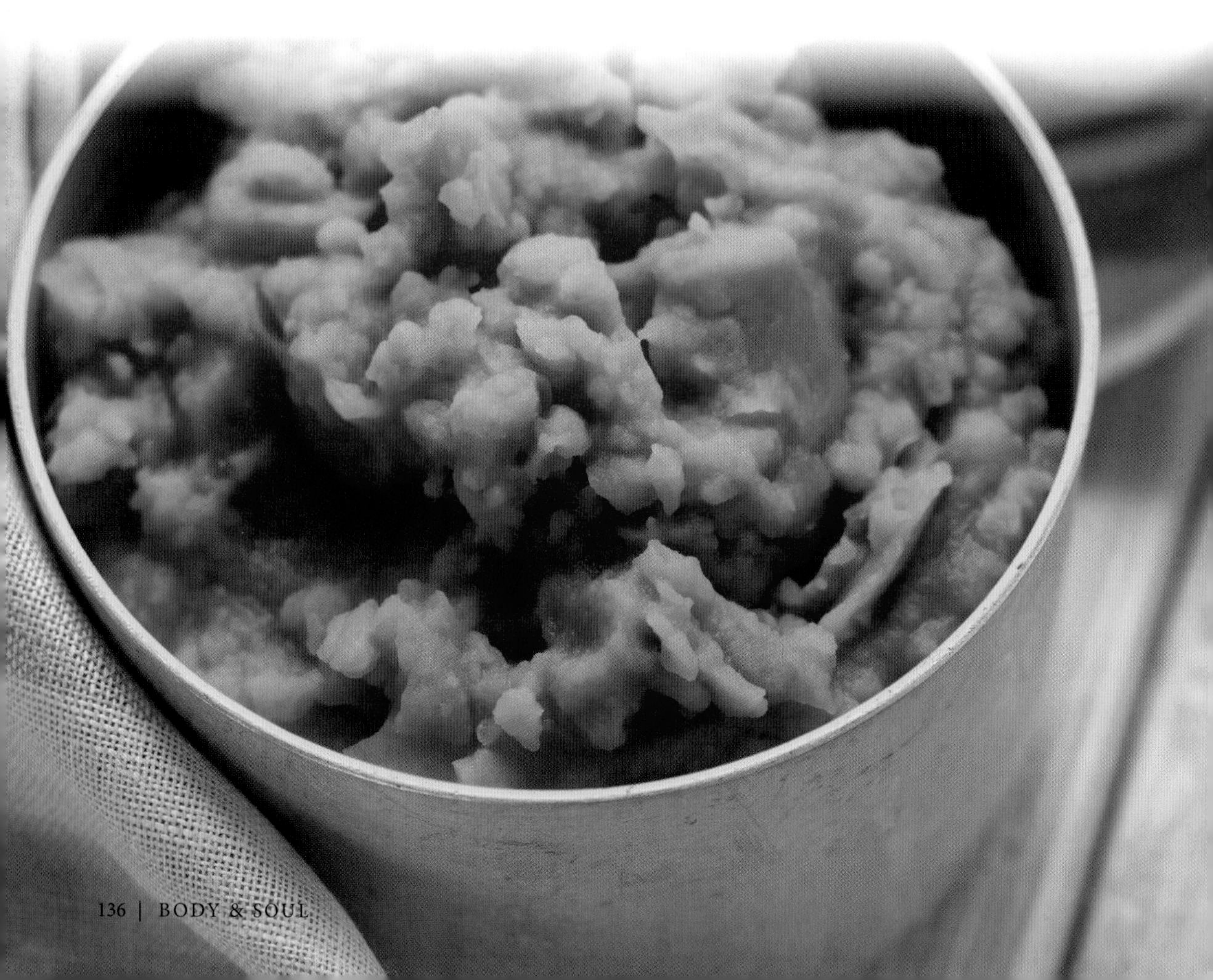

GREEN BASIL PESTO

This isn't exactly a side dish, but it is great for dipping veggies into or putting on top of crackers. Basil is full of nutrients, so it's way better for you than ranch dressing. This is my signature dip!

- 2 cups nuts (macadamia, cashews, or walnuts)
- 1/2 cup raw pumpkin seeds
- 1 bunch of basil
- 2 garlic cloves, peeled
- Sea salt and freshly ground black pepper to taste
- Chili flakes (if you like a dash of spice)
- 1/2 to 1 cup olive oil

Put all ingredients, except oil, in a food processor and mix. Slowly add oil while processor is running. Pesto should be thoroughly mixed but not too liquid-y.

I love to grow basil in my garden. Then I pick the leaves to make different versions of this delicious pesto.

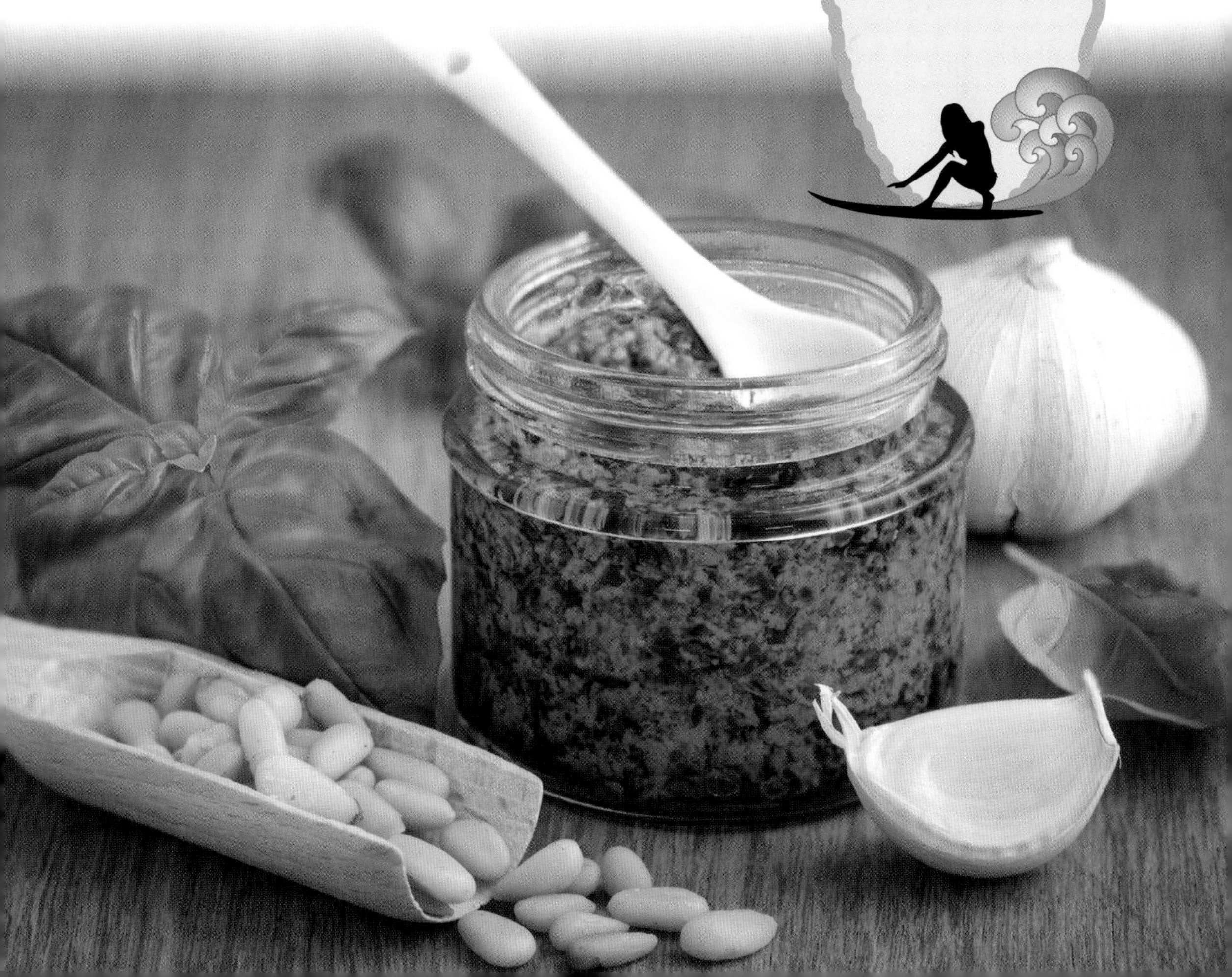

Desserts and Snacks

You might be committed to eating right, but you don't have to skip the sweets—just pick better-for-you ones and you'll satisfy those cravings in a second. Like salty? We've got a treat for you too.

COCONUT CHIA SEED PUDDING

Chia seeds are crazy good for you and available in all health food stores (and, increasingly, normal grocery stores). Make it your mission to give these petite powerhouse seeds a try. In pudding, they're unbeatable.

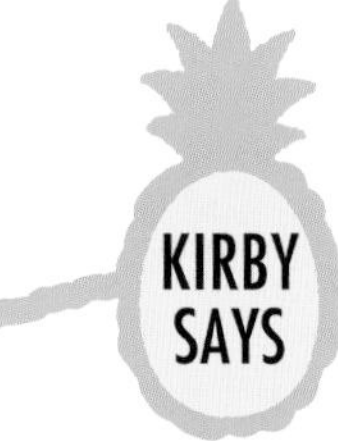

This pudding is so healthy, you can actually eat it at breakfast. Starting the day with dessert? Sounds good to me.

SERVES 2

1 cup organic coconut milk

1/4 cup chia seeds

1 tbsp. local honey (or to taste)

Handful of fruit

Mix all ingredients in a bowl and chill for at least 2 hours. Don't worry, the chia seeds will firm up a bit while in the fridge. Top with blueberries or any fruit of your choice.

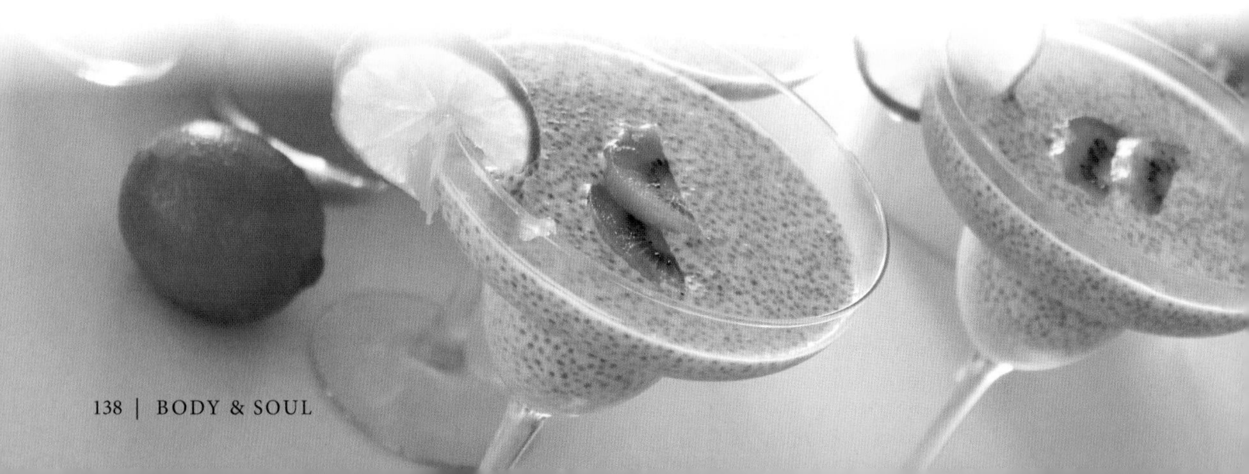

KALE CHIPS

Your soon-to-be-favorite leafy green bakes up to a mean chip. Plus, they cook in almost no time.

---

3 to 4 kale leaves, washed

1 tbsp. coconut oil

1 tsp. your favorite seasoned sea salt (just be sure it doesn't have any MSG!)

Preheat oven to 375°F. Dry kale with a paper towel. Remove the ribs from the kale by carefully ripping the leaves or cutting them. Cut the leaves into small pieces (but not too mini!). Put the leaves in a bowl and drizzle with oil; stir to coat each leaf. Line a baking sheet with parchment paper. Spread out the kale, making sure the leaves don't touch. Sprinkle on seasoning salt and bake for 12 minutes, or until crispy. (Check every few minutes, so they don't burn.)

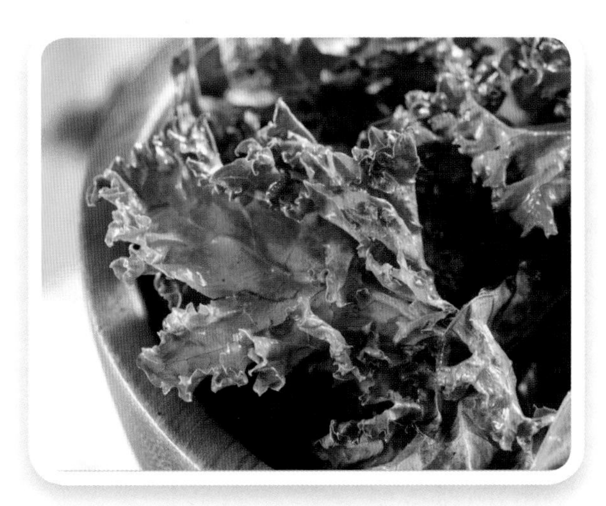

BANANA "ICE CREAM" 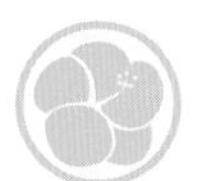

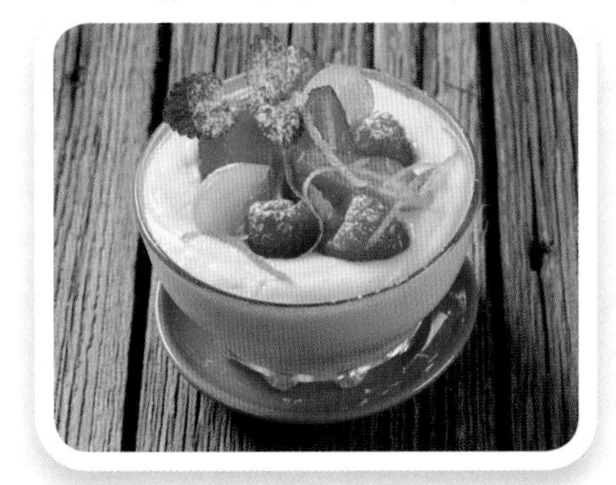

This dessert is sweet, creamy, and the perfect way to end your night. You might never go for the real stuff again—well, maybe.

SERVES 1

1 ripe banana (frozen), peeled and chopped

1/4 cup coconut milk

1 tbsp. sliced almonds (optional)

1 pinch shredded organic coconut (optional)

Puree banana in the blender; add coconut milk. Top with almonds and shredded coconut. You can add basically anything—frozen cherries, strawberries, dark chocolate, or whatever you like.

GOOD-FOR-YOU APPLE PIE

Pure Americana in each healthy bite, but the date crust gives it a major nutritious spin.

SERVES 8-12, DEPENDING ON HOW YOU SLICE IT

FOR THE APPLE FILLING:

1 cup raisins

8 to 9 organic apples (go for Gala if you want it sweet or Granny Smith if you want it a little tart)

2 tbsp. ground flaxseed

2 tsp. ground cinnamon

1/2 tsp. allspice

FOR THE PIECRUST:

2 cups chopped dates

1 cup raw almonds

1 cup raw cashews or hazelnuts

Zest of 1 orange

Juice from 1/4 orange

Pour some water into a small saucepan. Heat on medium-high until water boils. Carefully place raisins in water. Heat for five minutes. Drain raisins, reserving liquids. Then rinse raisins under cold water.

Core apples and chop into medium pieces. Mix half the apples in the food processor with the remaining ingredients until smooth, including the remaining reserved liquid the raisins were soaked in. Set aside in bowl. Mix remaining apples in the food processor, leaving chunks for texture. Mix the chunky apples with the smooth mixture.

Put piecrust ingredients into food processor and pulse. With hands, work into a dough and press into a 9-inch pie pan. Add the filling, and that's it. (You don't bake this pie, which is why it's sometimes dubbed a "live pie.").

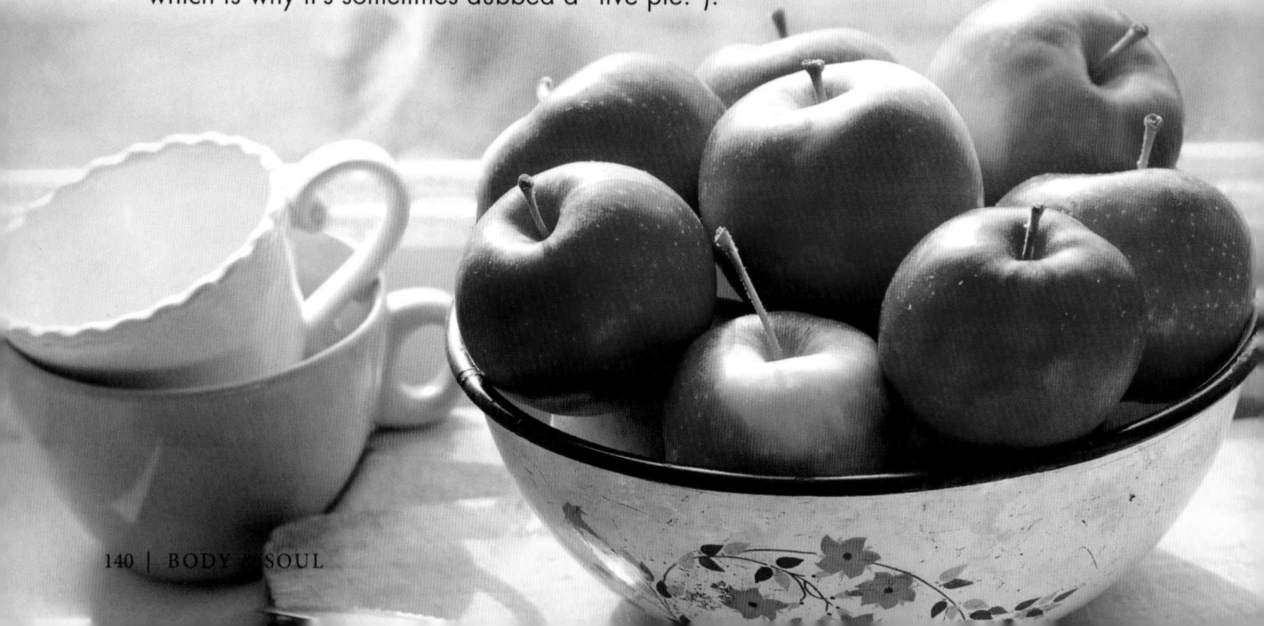

FROZEN YOGURT-COVERED BLUEBERRIES

This recipe is awesome. You can also add honey or vanilla yogurt and strawberries. All taste great.

SERVES 2

3/4 cup organic fresh blueberries

3/4 cup blueberry Greek yogurt (1 6-ounce container)

Wash blueberries and line a small baking sheet with parchment or waxed paper. Using a toothpick, dip each blueberry into the Greek yogurt and swirl until the blueberry is nicely coated with yogurt. Place on prepared baking sheet. Continue until all blueberries are coated. Place baking sheet in the freezer for at least 1 hour.

After 1 hour, the berries can be placed in a glass container and stored in the freezer. Take out what you need for snack time and enjoy.

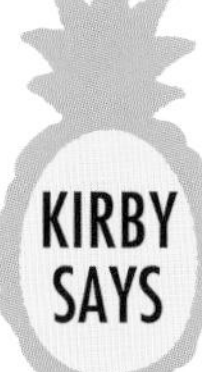

KIRBY SAYS

If you are lactose intolerant, enjoy frozen blueberries with unsweetened almond milk.

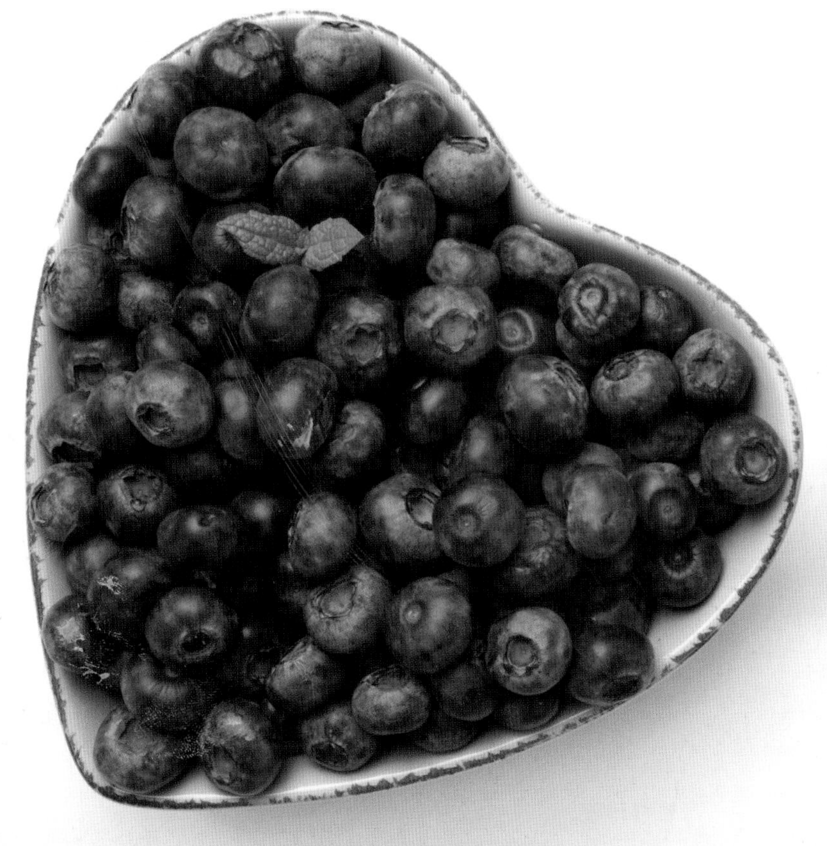

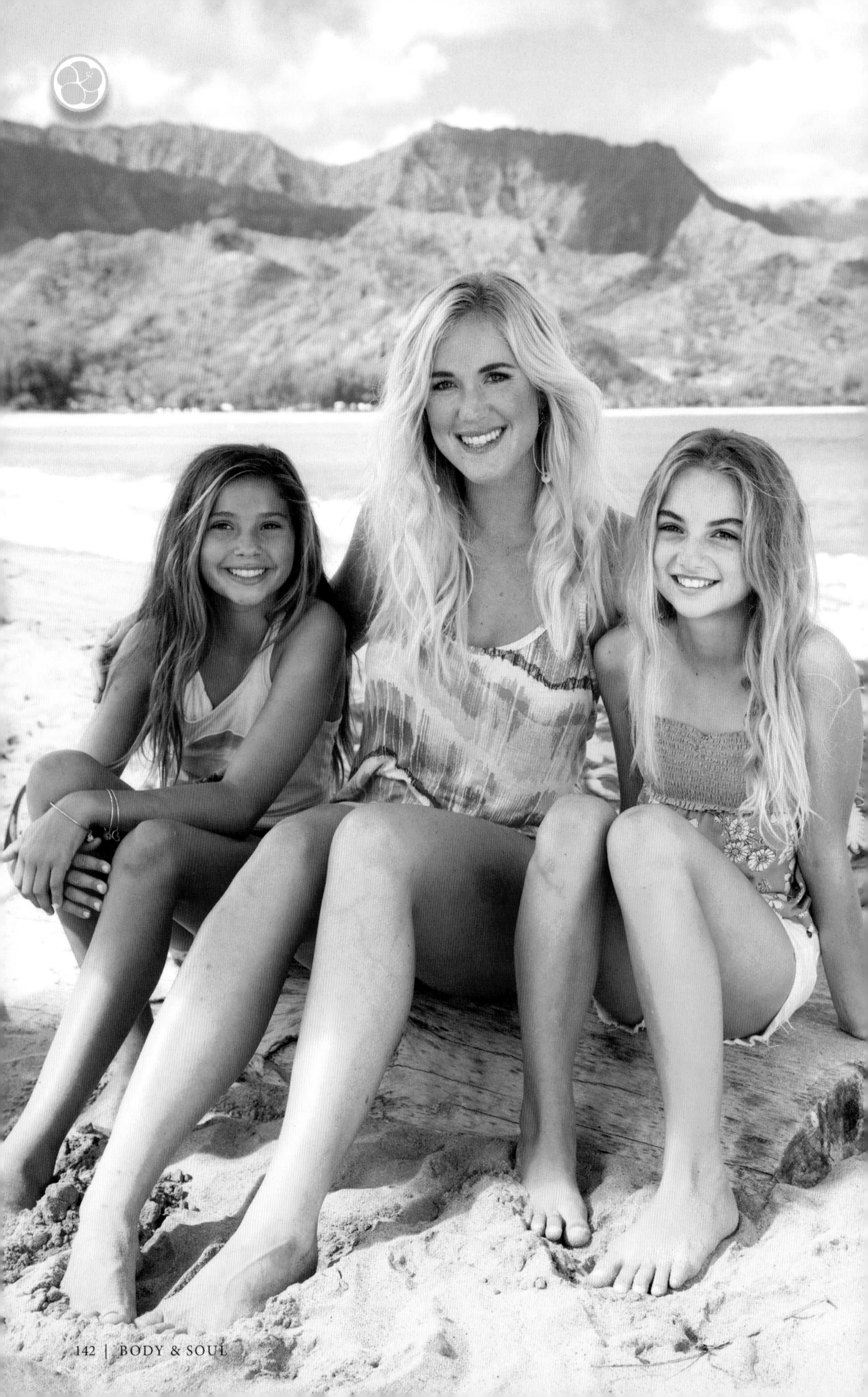

CHAPTER 9

Your Perfect Plan

So where to start? Right here, girl. I've whipped up a week showing you exactly what to eat, drink, and do to reveal your healthiest body and happiest self. After these seven days, I'll bet you'll feel amazing and be totally proud of what you've accomplished.

Remember: Don't feel bad if you're craving cookies like crazy or decide to have pizza for dinner one night. Change takes time, and jumping in with two feet isn't the right approach for everyone. Just do what feels right and wake up every morning thanking God, remembering you have the power to make your day great.

Psst. New to working out and eating right? Check in with your doctor first to make sure you're A-OK to start the plan.

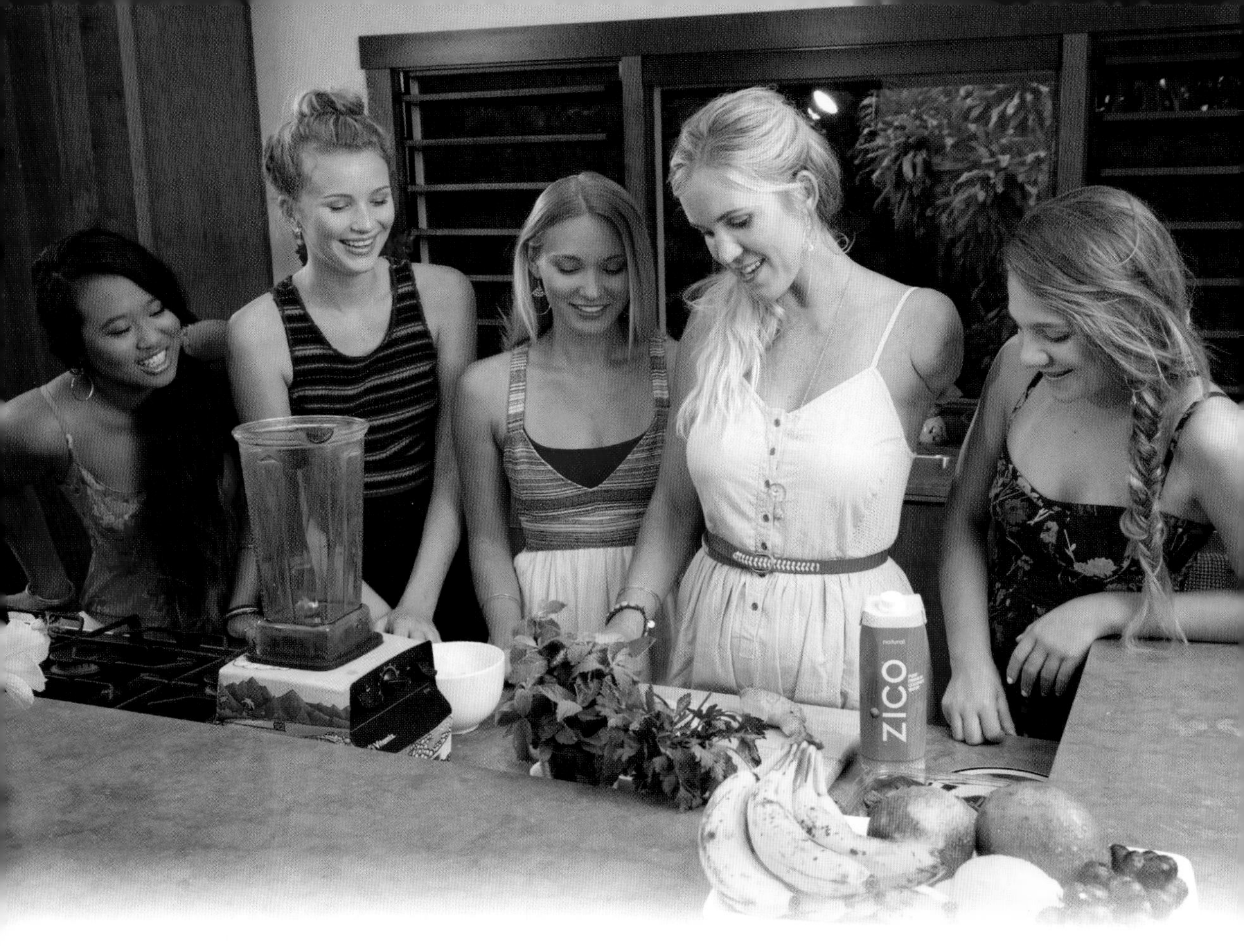

YOUR PERFECT PLAN FOR THE WEEK

Sunday

The day of rest also happens to be a great time to get in a long, slow workout, relax with your friends, go to church, grocery shop, and get prepped (mentally and physically) for the rest of the week.

8:00 a.m. WAKE UP!

Spend a few extra minutes in bed to stretch and say a quick prayer. Then pop on your slippers and get to the kitchen. Drink a big glass of water with lemon.

8:30 a.m. BREAKFAST

Take a head count of who's in the house and make some baked kale chips (page139). If you have a friend over, ask her to make P.O.G. juice (page 116). If not, brew some herbal tea for you and your family.

11:00 a.m. SNACK

Have something simple like apples and almond butter. If you have extra time, make kale chips (page 139) and mango muffins (page107) for later.

1:00 p.m. LUNCH

Time for some chicken nori wraps (page 119).

Pro Tip: Save the extra chicken for tomorrow's salad.

3:00 or 4:00 p.m. SNACK

If you've already gotten your workout in, refuel with a mango ginger smoothie (page 113).

6:00 or 7:00 p.m. DINNER

Grilled fish (try the recipe on page 126) with a side, like purple sweet potatoes (page 136).

Before 8:00 p.m. DESSERT

Go nuts with some banana "ice cream" (page 139). Drizzle with a little honey or top with a few dark chocolate chips.

DAILY WORKOUT

Sundays feel just right for a hike with your friends, a long bike ride, or yoga. Try something that will clear your head and help you feel refreshed going into the school week. It's also helpful to write down your goals at the start of the week, so break out the pen and paper. Dream and plan out what you want to achieve in the next few days

---

Monday

Everyone is on a different schedule for school, so I'm not going to even try to guess what time you get up, take lunch breaks, make time for snacks, etc. Instead, aim to eat every few hours and stay hydrated. In the morning, try to spend a few minutes being mindful (either praying or doing some deep breathing or both!) and, at the end of the day, don't eat too close to bedtime.

BREAKFAST

Mango muffins (you made them yesterday) and a green smoothie (page 114).

SNACK

Water, plus a Greek yogurt and a piece of fruit.

LUNCH

Greek theme salad (page 122), topped with the leftover chicken from yesterday's lunch. For a sweet finish, have some sliced pineapple.

SNACK

A handful of your favorite nuts, plus some veggies with pesto (if you're still hungry).

DINNER

Ahi poke bowl (page 120), with veggie quinoa (page 135) on the side. **Hint:** Make at least an extra cup of quinoa—you'll see why soon.

DESSERT

Chia seed pudding (page 138). Make extra, trust me! Or create an avocado smoothie.

DAILY WORKOUT

Super Stability workout (page 64), plus some stretching.

Tuesday

It's still the beginning of the week, so you likely have lots of energy. To help your future self (that's you on Thursday!), spend some time tonight making tasty snacks you'll want to eat later on those big temptation days.

BREAKFAST

Quinoa bowl (page 135), topped with fruit and nuts. Herbal tea on the side.

SNACK

Leftover mango muffin.

LUNCH

To-go salad (page 122) wrapped in a nori sheet. Your choice on the salad.

SNACK

Apples and almond butter or a Greek yogurt with an apple.

DINNER

Taco salad (page 122) and guacamole (page 132).

DESSERT

A couple squares of dark chocolate and a piece of fruit.

DAILY WORKOUT

It's cardio time. Aim for 30 minutes of running, biking, walking, dancing, or swimming.

BETHANY TIP: This evening, try making summer rolls (page121), so you can have a fun lunch tomorrow. If you have five extra minutes, try making the yogurt-covered berries (page 141).

Wednesday

You're halfway through the week, so check in with how you're feeling as soon as you wake up. Take a few minutes to write in your journal about how you're doing on your journey so far. Maybe you're overwhelmed, which might be a good sign to take today off from a tough workout, or (maybe) a little extra cardio today is just what you need to blast the anxiety.

BREAKFAST

Chia seed pudding and a piece of fruit. Start drinking your water early.

SNACK

Treat yourself to a green smoothie (bring it to school in a thermos).

LUNCH

Summer rolls with apple slices and almond butter on the side.

SNACK

Kale chips (page 137) and hummus, or cut veggies and pesto (page 137).

DINNER

Macadamia-crusted chicken (page125) with oven-roasted asparagus (page 134). Feel free to substitute other veggies, if you prefer.

DESSERT

Yogurt-covered berries (page 141) and some vanilla herbal tea.

DAILY WORKOUT

Do Dustin's "Posture Up!" moves (page 70).

Thursday

Take a few deep inhales and exhales as soon as you rise and shine. Later in the week, it can be hard to stay committed to your plan. Start the day with eggs to really energize you and then keep a positive attitude throughout school. When you're done? Nix stress with some intense cardio. You're almost there!

BREAKFAST

Make an inside-out omlette (page 111) and drink tons of water or green tea.

SNACK

Greek yogurt and fruit gives you some sweetness plus protein.

LUNCH

Rock a big salad with some leftover chicken from last night.

Hint: Cut up extra veggies in the a.m. when you're whipping up those eggs.

SNACK

Treat yourself to your favorite smoothie. This time get creative with the ingredients.

DINNER

Grilled chicken or fish with your favorite veggie side (cook's choice).

DESSERT

A couple squares of dark chocolate or leftover yogurt-covered berries.

DAILY WORKOUT

It's a cardio day but don't be afraid to go hard.
Try intervals or an intense cardio class at the gym.

BETHANY TIP: Make some quinoa or chia seed pudding tonight, so you're ready for tomorrow's breakfast.

Friday

The weekend is almost here, girl. Start the day by doing some stretching in bed or a couple of yoga poses before you have breakfast. After working out all week, you're bound to be a little sore. Stay hydrated and happy.

BREAKFAST

A green smoothie and the quinoa or chia pudding you made last night, topped with fruit.

SNACK

Celery and almond butter or some nuts and a piece of fruit.

LUNCH

Go for an all-veggie salad (page 122) topped with some seeds, nuts, or beans.

SNACK

Time for your fave healthy-girl snack: trail mix, fruit, a smoothie, yogurt, kale chips, or whatever you love.

DINNER

Invite a couple friends over and make something together. Theme salads, perhaps?

DESSERT

Banana ice cream (page 139) with your BFFs. Turn it into a sundae bar, with a few healthy toppings to choose from. (Try organic coconut shreds, dark chocolate chips, sliced almonds, and cherries or strawberries in season. Want a tasty treat? Sprinkle on a little cinnamon.)

DAILY WORKOUT:

"Awesome Agility" (page 74) and then some stretching.

Saturday

By now, eating right is nothing new. But the weekend presents special challenges, with people pigging out all over the place. A week in, though, you're probably feeling pretty amazing, after all that eating clean and working out. While it's tempting to cave today, stay committed to your plan. Tomorrow, you'll be thrilled you did.

BREAKFAST

Whichever egg and kale recipe you love best. Have some tea too.

SNACK

Get out the blender and make no-banana smoothie (page 112).

LUNCH

You pick! Whatever good-for-you foods you're craving, go for it.

SNACK

Yogurt with honey, berries, and nuts. Put it in a fancy glass for a fun parfait.

DINNER

Play around with a tapas-style dinner, serving a few small versions of your favorites, like summer rolls, purple sweet potatoes, and a Caesar salad.

DESSERT

Make some muffins since you've got extra time. This time try replacing the mango (page 107) with something else, like blackberries.

DAILY WORKOUT:

Just play. Do whatever active thing you absolutely love, whether it's shooting hoops or practicing yoga. It's Saturday, so have fun and give yourself a big high-five for your first week of eating clean and treating your body with total respect.

WHAT TO SKIP

It can seem overwhelming to wrap your head around, but added chemicals in foods just aren't good for you. To help you keep an eye out for those sneaky ingredients, Kirby came up with a list of additives to avoid. Fresh is always best, and guess what? None of these bad ingredients are in organic fruits, vegetables, eggs, fish, or meats.

Ingredient: Artificial Sweeteners like Aspartame (Equal, NutraSweet), Sucralose (Splenda), Neotame, Saccharin (Sweet 'N' Low), and Acesulfame Potassium (sometimes called Sweet One).

Found in: "Diet" products, low-fat foods, and anything that is way sweet but is boasting low calories.

Why it's bad: Each of these sweeteners potentially cause problems with your nervous system, like headaches or dizziness, and some may even cause cancer in animals.

Ingredient: High-Fructose Corn Syrup

Found in: Soda, candy, packaged desserts, and much, much more.

Why it's bad: It can lead to obesity, increased belly fat, and heart disease.

Ingredient: Preservatives like polysorbates, nitrites, nitrates, sulfites, TBHQ, BHT, BHA, potassium sorbate, and sodium benzoate.

Found in: Packaged foods, deli meats, juice, and much more.

Why it's bad: Designed to make foods last longer, this group often causes people to have allergic reactions, nausea, and vomiting. Some of the more serious health problems include messing with your body at the DNA level, as well as liver or kidney issues.

Ingredient: Artificial Flavorings and Coloring (this is a blanket term for over 100 possible additives).

Found in: Lots of foods that sit on the shelf for a while, like drinks, crackers, or any food that is flavored like something else.

Why it's bad: These can cause behavioral problems or allergic reactions.

Ingredient: Monosodium Glutamate a.k.a. MSG

Found in: Processed foods, like frozen dinners, chips, condiments, and candies.

Why it's bad: It can leave people with chest pains, heart palpitations and headaches. Plus, it can stimulate your taste buds, so you crave more food, even right after eating.

Ingredient: Trans Fats like shortening, partially hydrogenated fats, monounsaturated fats, and diglycerides, or DATEM.

Found in: Store-bought baked goods, salad dressings, ice cream and much, much more.

Why it's bad: This group of bad fats can leave people with heart disease, cancer, or diabetes.

EQUIVALENTS AND METRIC CONVERSIONS

The following figures are approximate metric weight and volume equivalents for common measurements provided in this cookbook. If converting to metric, use the volume amount when the U.S. measurement is given by volume (teaspoon, tablespoon, cup), and use the weight equivalent when the U.S. measurement is given by weight (ounce, pound).

U.S. Measurement	Metric Equivalent
¼ cup	60 milliliters
⅓ cup	80 milliliters
½ cup	120 milliliters
1 cup	8 fluid ounces or 236 milliliters
2 cups	460 milliliters
1 tablespoon	.5 fluid ounce or 14.8 milliliters
1 teaspoon	4.9 milliliters
1 ounce	28.35 grams
1 pound	453.59 grams
¼ inch	.6 centimeters
1 inch	2.5 centimeters

For metric equivalents, use the following general formulas:

- Ounces to grams — multiply ounces by 28.35
- Pounds to grams — multiply pounds by 453.5
- Pounds to kilograms — multiply pounds by .45
- Cups to liters — multiply cups by .24
- Fahrenheit to centigrade — subtract 32 from Fahrenheit temperature, multiply by 5, then divide by 9

The following equivalents will help you when you need to double or half a recipe.

Measurement	Equivalent
1 tablespoon	3 teaspoons
¼ cup	4 tablespoons or 12 teaspoons
½ cup	8 tablespoons
1 pint	2 cups
1 cup	8 fluid ounces
1 quart	4 cups

AFTERWORD

I'm so, so, so proud of you for doing your best! Remember, if you fall off your surfboard, get back on and keep trying. Or in surf terms, "keep ripping!"

Track your progress using a journal or an online app (there are lots out there). Write how you feel about your body and mind changing. Take note of your energy levels and how you feel. Also note improvements in your skin, hair, and nails. Keep learning and investigating. Sometimes when I try a new food, say cilantro in my salad, I'll look up cilantro to see what its nutritional benefits are. Never stop educating yourself about good health. Try new recipes and workouts. Stay motivated by trying new moves and including friends or family. Keep pushing yourself. Continue your spiritual journey, building your relationship with Jesus Christ, so you can maintain perspective on what is most important in life. Remember, Jesus loves you just as you are, so HAVE FUN and just BE YOUR BEAUTIFUL SELF!

For more healthy recipes and tips, visit my website, BethanyHamilton.com, where you can sign up for my monthly newsletter for more updates and ideas.

Aloha!

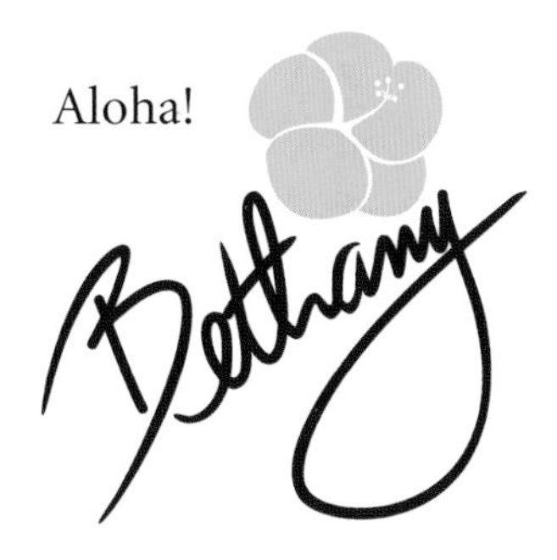

Thank you to everyone at Zondervan who worked so hard on this book:
Kim Childress, Cindy Davis, Kris Nelson, Diane Mielke, Nan Snow,
Annette Bourland, Sara Merritt, Chriscynethia Floyd, and Ashley Willis.

And thanks to my great team, including my writers:
Katie Abbondanza, Sarah Wassner Flynn, and Patricia McNamara.

Thanks to Sean Scheidt for the fabulous photos in this book,
Jessica D'Argenio Waller for the amazing styling,
and Leah Bassett for the gorgeous hair and makeup.
And to Karen Bokram for bringing it all together.

INTERESTED IN GROWING YOUR FAITH?

Here are some great books from Bethany Hamilton in the

Soul Surfer Series

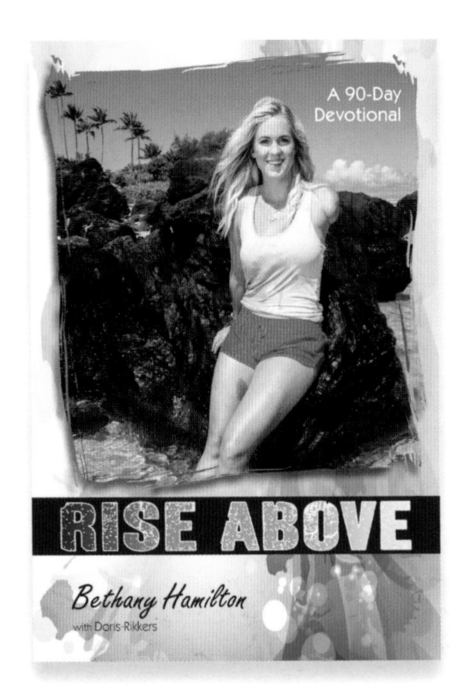

Rise Above

A 90-Day Devotional

Author: Bethany Hamilton with Doris Rikkers

Bethany Hamilton shares with young girls her courage and enthusiasm for God, inspiring them to face life head on and stand strong in their faith.

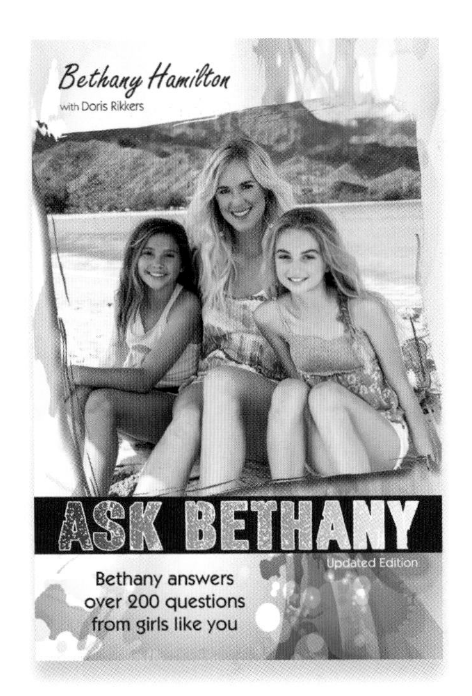

Ask Bethany, Updated Edition

Bethany answers over 200 questions from girls like you

Author: Bethany Hamilton with Doris Rikkers

From Bethany Hamilton's fan letters come these honest, sometimes gut-wrenching questions—probably questions you've asked. Verses from the Bible add inspiration to Bethany's sincere answers.